Heartbreak Book for Women

CRAFTED BY SKRIUWER

Copyright © 2024 by Skriuwer.

All rights reserved. No part of this book may be used or reproduced in any form whatsoever without written permission except in the case of brief quotations in critical articles or reviews.

For more information, contact : **kontakt@skriuwer.com** (www.skriuwer.com)

TABLE OF CONTENTS

CHAPTER 1: WHAT HEARTBREAK MEANS

- Explains the depth of heartbreak and why it feels overwhelming
- Discusses cultural and personal factors that make heartbreak intense
- Highlights physical signs that show heartbreak is more than just "in the head"

CHAPTER 2: HOW HEARTBREAK AFFECTS THOUGHTS AND EMOTIONS

- Shows the common thought patterns that accompany heartbreak
- Offers ways to cope with sadness, anger, and confusion
- Suggests practical strategies for reducing rumination

CHAPTER 3: PHYSICAL EFFECTS OF SADNESS

- Covers how heartbreak can lead to real bodily symptoms
- Explores basic methods to handle fatigue, pain, and poor sleep
- Emphasizes the importance of caring for the body during emotional distress

CHAPTER 4: COMMON MISTAKES PEOPLE MAKE AFTER A BREAKUP

- Identifies typical traps (like rebound relationships or social media drama)
- Warns against self-sabotage and substance reliance
- Provides healthier alternatives to move forward responsibly

CHAPTER 5: HEALTHY WAYS TO EXPRESS SAD FEELINGS

- Describes safe outlets for emotional release (art, journaling, support)
- Teaches the difference between bottling up and constructive sharing
- Offers simple exercises to reduce emotional overload

CHAPTER 6: DEALING WITH LOSS OF SELF-WORTH

- Explores how heartbreak can damage self-esteem
- Proposes methods for regaining confidence step by step
- Introduces ways to replace negative self-talk with kinder perspectives

CHAPTER 7: SELF-CARE BASICS FOR EMOTIONAL PAIN

- Lays out daily routines that support healing
- Explains the role of consistent habits in rebuilding stability
- Provides tips for setting up a balanced self-care schedule

CHAPTER 8: HOW TO ASK FOR HELP AND SUPPORT

- Offers scripts and suggestions for reaching out to friends or professionals
- Highlights the importance of vulnerability balanced with self-respect
- Shows ways to accept help without feeling like a burden

CHAPTER 9: REBUILDING TRUST IN YOURSELF

- Details how heartbreak can damage self-confidence
- Introduces small exercises to restore belief in personal decisions
- Teaches the value of assertiveness and clear thinking

CHAPTER 10: LEARNING FROM PAST EXPERIENCES

- Advises on reviewing past relationships without getting stuck in regret
- Discusses patterns and lessons that can prevent repeated heartbreak
- Suggests reflective methods for healthier future connections

CHAPTER 11: CONFIDENCE-BUILDING PRACTICES

- Suggests routines to solidify self-esteem (positive self-talk, posture tips)
- Explains the link between personal accomplishments and emotional recovery
- Encourages small, consistent wins to strengthen self-view

CHAPTER 12: COMMUNICATION TIPS FOR FUTURE RELATIONSHIPS

- Discusses assertive yet empathetic conversation strategies
- Emphasizes active listening and boundary-setting in new bonds
- Teaches how to avoid misunderstandings rooted in past heartbreak

CHAPTER 13: HANDLING SINGLE LIFE AFTER HEARTBREAK

- Suggests ways to cope with loneliness and redefine daily routines
- Explores the upsides of being single, including personal growth
- Encourages reconnecting with old friends and trying new hobbies

CHAPTER 14: MANAGING SOCIAL PRESSURES

- Explains how family and friends can unknowingly add breakup stress
- Presents tactics for politely declining intrusive questions
- Teaches self-assertion in the face of cultural or social expectations

CHAPTER 15: NURTURING NEW FRIENDSHIPS

- Highlights the value of non-romantic bonds for emotional support
- Gives tips for meeting people, from casual chats to group activities
- Describes maintaining healthy boundaries in emerging friendships

CHAPTER 16: HANDLING ANGER AND RESENTMENT

- Clarifies the difference between anger and long-term resentment
- Shares outlets for safe emotional release
- Offers strategies for letting go of grudges and finding closure

CHAPTER 17: FINANCIAL INDEPENDENCE AND EMOTIONAL FREEDOM

- Links money stability to reduced breakup anxiety
- Covers budgeting basics, debt management, and setting financial goals
- Explains how financial control reinforces personal confidence

CHAPTER 18: SETTING CLEAR BOUNDARIES

- Defines emotional, physical, and digital boundaries for well-being
- Teaches how to communicate limits assertively but respectfully
- Guides on handling pushback from ex-partners, family, or friends

CHAPTER 19: FINDING PURPOSE OUTSIDE ROMANTIC LOVE

- Explores diverse life areas (career, hobbies, friendships) as sources of meaning
- Suggests methods for creating personal mission statements
- Discusses how heartbreak can open new avenues of self-discovery

CHAPTER 20: MOVING FORWARD WITH HOPE AND STRENGTH

- Summarizes ways to accept change while avoiding cynicism
- Emphasizes building long-term resilience with healthy routines
- Concludes with a focus on ongoing growth and the bright possibilities ahead

Chapter 1: What Heartbreak Means

Heartbreak is a deep feeling of loss that happens when someone we care about is no longer in our lives in the same way. It can happen when a romantic relationship ends or when trust is broken. It can make a person feel worthless, lonely, or confused. Women of all ages can feel it. It is not a small issue. It can feel like a huge shift in life that affects everything around us.

Heartbreak is often linked with a breakup, but it can also happen when you learn that someone you love is not who you thought they were, or when you lose a friend or face another form of loss. The emotions can be powerful, and it can be hard to know how to handle them.

In many cultures, there is an unspoken rule that a person should just get over a breakup. But heartbreak is not just about missing someone. It can shake your sense of safety, your understanding of love, and your overall view of the future. Heartbreak can also remind you of other losses you have faced in life, which can make it feel even bigger.

Some people think that heartbreak is only emotional, but it can cause physical symptoms too. You might feel headaches, loss of appetite, or even unexplained aches in your body. This is because our minds and bodies work together. When your thoughts are sad or stressed, your body can react in many ways.

Different Forms of Heartbreak

- **Sudden Breakup**: This happens when a partner decides to end the relationship without much warning. It can be shocking, causing confusion and disbelief. The person left behind might feel they had no chance to fix things or discuss what went wrong.
- **Gradual Drift**: This is when two people slowly grow apart. The breakup might be mutual, but it can still be hurtful. Women might feel upset that the excitement has faded or that their partner no longer values them in the same way.
- **Betrayal**: This can happen when someone finds out their partner was not loyal. The feeling of betrayal can be a deep wound that stays for a long time, making a person question their worth and their ability to trust.
- **Unrequited Feelings**: This heartbreak happens when you care about someone, but they do not feel the same way. Even though there might not

have been a clear relationship, it still hurts to face the loss of hope and the sting of rejection.

Why Women Feel It Strongly

Heartbreak can be painful for anyone, but some women experience it with extra intensity due to social and cultural factors. In many societies, women are taught from a young age to place importance on relationships and emotional connection. They might feel pressure to be perfect partners or caregivers. When a relationship ends, it can feel like they have failed or let others down.

Women sometimes put their own goals on hold for the sake of a relationship. They might move to a new place to be with a partner, or they might stop focusing on their personal growth because they believe love is the most important part of life. When things end, they can feel lost, unsure of how to move forward.

The Weight of Expectations

Expectations can make heartbreak heavier. A woman might have pictured a certain path: marriage, children, a shared home, and a long life with a partner. When the relationship ends, all these hopes can vanish at once. This can create a feeling of grief not just for the person but for the future plans that now feel impossible.

Society can also add pressure by questioning a woman's single status. Some people ask, "When are you getting married?" or, "Why aren't you dating?" These questions can cause more stress and make a woman feel like she is not living up to what others want.

The Difference Between Sadness and Heartbreak

Sadness is a common emotion that appears from time to time. Heartbreak is deeper. It is a kind of sadness tied to loss, whether real or imagined. Sadness might come and go, but heartbreak can linger and affect everyday life for a longer period. It might change how a person sees themselves, leading to thoughts like, "I'm not lovable," or, "I am not important anymore."

Overcoming Shame

Many women feel ashamed after heartbreak. They might think they did something to cause the breakup, or they may feel weak for not being able to move on quickly. Shame can feed on isolation. When a person hides their heartbreak, they have no space to discuss their feelings in a healthy way.

It is important to understand that heartbreak is not a sign of weakness. It is a sign that you cared about someone. Feeling sad is not the problem; refusing to address it is what can create long-term issues. If you pretend the pain is not there, it can grow into bigger emotional hurdles.

The Impact on Identity

When people are in relationships, their sense of self might become closely tied to their partner. Some people center their daily life around the other person's schedule, likes, and dislikes. Over time, they might forget their own needs and hobbies. After a breakup, they might suddenly wonder, "Who am I without my partner?"

This loss of identity can make heartbreak more painful. It is not only about losing a person; it is about losing a version of yourself that existed in that relationship. You might have to discover or rediscover who you are and what you want from life.

The Importance of Real Talk

Some friends and family members might say well-intentioned things like, "You will be fine," or "Just forget about it." While they might be trying to help, these phrases can shut down honest discussion of the pain. It is okay to talk about your true feelings. It can be helpful to speak with a trusted friend or counselor who will listen without judging.

Having real talk helps you see that heartbreak is a real experience that calls for real attention. It is not just a small bump in the road. It deserves understanding and kindness.

Social Media Traps

In today's world, heartbreak can become even more painful because of social media. You might be tempted to check your ex-partner's online posts, or you might see pictures of them having fun. This can add more pain. Constant reminders of their presence, or seeing them with new people, can make the healing process slower.

A helpful approach is to limit social media use during this time or block or mute the ex-partner's accounts. This small step can protect your mind from extra harm. It might feel tough at first, but it can make a big difference in how quickly you start to feel better.

Uncommon Information to Remember

- **Brain Chemistry Factor**: Research shows that heartbreak can light up the same areas of the brain that respond to physical pain. This is why emotional pain feels so intense. It is not your imagination. Your brain is literally signaling that something hurts.
- **Repetitive Thinking**: Some women get stuck in loops of negative thoughts, often wondering if they could have changed things or if they will ever find someone better. Setting aside a short time each day to write thoughts on paper can prevent these loops from taking over. This might allow for a calmer mind after finishing the writing exercise.
- **Boundary Setting for Self**: It is not just about setting limits with others. You might need to set limits with your own behaviors. This could mean telling yourself, "I will not check their social media for at least two weeks," and sticking to that promise. This is a way to protect your own healing process.

First Steps to Cope

1. **Allow the Tears**: Crying can release tension and reduce stress. It can help your body let go of built-up emotions. There is nothing wrong with crying.
2. **Share with Someone Trustworthy**: If you have a friend who listens without trying to fix your emotions, talk to them. Speak plainly about how you feel.
3. **Do Not Blame Yourself Right Away**: It is common to think, "If only I had done this differently." But blame can trap you in guilt. Wait until you are calmer before reflecting on what went wrong.
4. **Keep a Simple Routine**: Basic daily tasks like making your bed and preparing a meal can provide a sense of stability. These small steps remind you that you can still accomplish things, even if you feel down.

5. **Try to Rest**: Heartbreak can interrupt sleep, but a stable sleep pattern can help your mind and body recover. If you struggle with rest, consider short breathing exercises before bed.

The Bigger Picture

This book will cover many parts of heartbreak. It will discuss how heartbreak affects thoughts, emotions, and even the body. It will go into practical steps for managing sadness and rebuilding confidence. It will also touch on how to avoid repeating the same mistakes in future connections.

It is important to keep in mind that you will not feel terrible forever. Emotions change over time. The end of a relationship can become the start of your personal growth. You can use this time to look at what went wrong, what you truly want, and how you can create a life that feels more true to who you are.

Conclusion of Chapter 1

Heartbreak is more than just a feeling of sadness. It can leave a person questioning their self-worth, their hopes, and their sense of stability. The weight of expectations and cultural norms can make it feel bigger. Understanding that it is normal to feel intense loss can be the first step to getting stronger. In the next chapter, we will discuss in detail how heartbreak affects your mind, from the thought patterns that pop up to the emotional waves that can come and go.

Chapter 2: How Heartbreak Affects Thoughts and Emotions

Heartbreak can bring up thoughts and emotions that seem to go in circles. You might be crying one moment, angry the next, and then feel numb or shocked soon after. This chapter explains why these emotional ups and downs happen. It will also address how your thoughts can become trapped in negative patterns. We will then look at steps you can take to free your mind and keep your emotions from controlling you.

Emotional Waves and Mood Changes

When heartbreak happens, the feelings do not arrive in a neat and orderly way. They can appear out of nowhere, even when you are busy doing something else. You might be folding clothes and suddenly remember a hurtful argument with your ex-partner. This memory can trigger sadness or anger.

- **Sadness and Grief**: These are the base emotions when dealing with heartbreak. You might cry without warning or feel a heavy weight in your chest. Grief can show itself through tears or by losing interest in activities you once enjoyed.
- **Anger and Blame**: Some women feel angry at their ex-partner or even at themselves. They might replay fights in their minds. Anger can give a burst of energy, but it can also lead to harmful decisions if not handled carefully.
- **Confusion**: After a breakup, you might not be sure why it happened or what led to the end. This confusion can cause restlessness. You might want to call your ex for answers, but sometimes the answers they give will not satisfy you, or they might not want to talk.
- **Numbness**: Some women feel so overwhelmed that they become numb. They do not cry or yell; they just feel empty. This does not mean the heartbreak is gone. It means the mind might be taking a break from all the strong feelings.
- **Relief**: In some cases, heartbreak can bring a strange sense of relief if the relationship was stressful. This relief might be mixed with guilt, making you wonder if you are a bad person for feeling okay about leaving a difficult situation.

Thought Patterns That Appear

1. **Overthinking**: You might play the same scenes in your head, wondering if you could have said something different or acted in another way. This overthinking can rob you of sleep and peace of mind.
2. **Self-Criticism**: During heartbreak, it is common to pick yourself apart. You might think, "I am not smart enough," or "I am not pretty enough," causing your confidence to drop.
3. **Fear of the Future**: You might worry that you will never find love again or that you are too old or too damaged to start over. This fear can be paralyzing.
4. **Denial**: Some people act like the breakup never happened. They refuse to accept it, which can delay healing. Denial can cause a person to hold onto a relationship that is already gone.
5. **Obsessing Over the Ex**: You might think about what your ex is doing all the time. This might include stalking them on social media or asking mutual friends about them. This is a natural urge but can lead to more pain.

How the Mind Responds to Loss

When you lose a relationship, the mind might treat it as if you lost a vital part of your life. The brain releases stress chemicals, like cortisol, when you feel threatened or anxious. Over time, high levels of stress hormones can make you feel constantly on edge, affecting your sleep and your ability to stay calm.

Also, emotional pain after heartbreak can feel as real as physical pain. Brain scans show that the same areas light up when a person goes through social rejection as when they feel actual physical pain. This means that heartbreak is not just "in your head" in the sense of it being imaginary. It has very real effects on the brain.

The Problem with Ruminating

Ruminating means thinking about the same bad thoughts again and again. When you ruminate, you hold onto a hurtful memory and keep replaying it. This can keep you trapped in the past and stop you from seeing any positive signs in your present life.

People often ruminate because they think they can find a solution if they think about it hard enough. But heartbreak rarely has a simple solution that appears through overthinking. Instead, ruminating can make you feel worse because it pushes you to focus on the pain.

Avoiding Unhelpful Coping Strategies

- **Drinking to Numb Feelings**: Some women might try to dull the pain with alcohol or other substances. While it can give short-term relief, the sadness often returns with more intensity.
- **Rebounding Immediately**: Jumping into another relationship right away can lead to problems. It might distract you briefly, but it does not address the root issues. You can carry old wounds into the new situation.
- **Venting Online**: Sometimes people post about their heartbreak on social media, hoping for attention or sympathy. This can cause more drama if the ex or mutual friends see it. It also makes it harder to heal in private.

Uncommon Facts About Thought and Emotion Control

1. **Cold Showers for Emotional Relief**: Research suggests that cold exposure (like a quick cold shower) can help reset the nervous system. It might reduce stress and help you think more clearly. While it will not solve heartbreak, it can give your mind a break from intense emotion.
2. **Chewing Gum to Distract the Brain**: A simple action like chewing gum can sometimes interrupt negative thought loops because you are engaging a part of the brain that deals with motor activity. It is not a cure, but it can help in the moment.
3. **Using 5-Minute Delays for Impulsive Actions**: If you feel the urge to send an angry text or call your ex, wait five minutes. This short delay can help you calm down and possibly make a better decision.

Naming Your Emotions

One way to handle emotional waves is to name them. For example, if you feel a rush of anger, say to yourself, "This is anger." If sadness comes over you, mentally say, "This is sadness." By naming the emotion, you create a small gap between the emotion and your response. This gap can help you control how you act.

Self-Compassion Techniques

- **Speak Kindly to Yourself**: Instead of calling yourself foolish or weak, try to speak to yourself as you would to a close friend. For instance, "I am in pain right now, and that's understandable."
- **Mirror Affirmations**: Stand in front of a mirror, look into your own eyes, and say something positive. It might feel strange at first, but it can gradually improve self-esteem.
- **Write a Letter to Yourself**: In this letter, acknowledge the hurt you feel. Also, write what you wish for yourself: peace, happiness, or hope. Read this letter when you feel overwhelmed.

Practical Ways to Keep Emotional Balance

1. **Daily Journaling**: Write a page or two each day about your thoughts. This helps you track your emotional shifts over time. You can see patterns and become more aware of changes in mood.
2. **Physical Activities**: Movement can help. Going for a walk, doing simple home exercises, or any activity that raises your heart rate can reduce stress chemicals. It also helps you sleep better at night.
3. **Scheduled Worry Time**: If you find yourself worrying all day, pick a specific 15-minute block during the day to let yourself worry. When those thoughts come up at other times, remind yourself that you have a scheduled time for them. This can help you manage anxious thoughts more efficiently.

Handling Emotional Overload at Work or in Public

Heartbreak does not stop when you leave home. It can follow you to work or social events. You might feel tears welling up in a meeting, or you might struggle to focus on tasks.

- **Short Breaks**: If you feel overwhelmed, excuse yourself for a few minutes. Go to the restroom, take a few slow breaths, and splash some cool water on your face.
- **Email Draft Method**: If you feel the urge to vent by sending an email or message, write it as a draft but do not send it. Wait until you have cooled down. Often, you will see that sending it might not help.
- **Visual Distractions**: Keep a family photo or a peaceful image on your desk. When you feel stressed, look at it for a moment. Try to focus on

details in the picture. This can help shift your mind away from distressing thoughts.

The Warning Signs of Deeper Emotional Issues

While heartbreak is normal, sometimes it can cause or worsen mental health issues. If you notice these signs, consider talking to a professional:

- Extreme mood swings that scare you
- Total loss of interest in daily tasks for weeks
- Frequent thoughts of harming yourself
- Uncontrolled anxiety that stops you from functioning

There is no shame in seeking help. A counselor or therapist can give you tools to manage strong emotions and thoughts more safely.

Avoiding Self-Fulfilling Worries

Sometimes women might think, "No one will ever love me again," or "I will always be alone." These are self-fulfilling if you believe them strongly. You might behave in ways that push people away, proving your fear right. Changing these negative beliefs early can prevent that cycle.

Moving From Emotional Reaction to Logical Action

Emotions are powerful, but life also requires day-to-day responsibilities. You might still have to work, take care of children, or pay bills. Here are some tips to help:

1. **Set Tiny Goals**: Instead of forcing yourself to act happy, set small tasks you can complete. This can be something like replying to emails or washing the dishes. Crossing small tasks off a list can give a sense of accomplishment.
2. **Plan for Emotional Outlets**: Schedule time for healthy outlets, such as talking with a friend or writing in a journal. Having a planned time for releasing feelings can help you focus on other tasks when needed.
3. **Use Support Systems**: Lean on friends or family for help with errands or babysitting if you have children. There is no prize for facing heartbreak alone.

Ways to Challenge Harmful Thoughts

- **Ask for Evidence**: If you think, "I am worthless," ask yourself, "Is there real evidence that I have no worth?" You will likely find many reasons why you do have value.
- **Think in Third Person**: Instead of saying, "I messed up," imagine a friend is in your situation. What would you say to them? This switch can help you see the situation in a more balanced way.
- **Use a Thought Record**: A simple chart where you write the situation, your thoughts, the emotions, and another possible viewpoint. This is a tool used in some therapy approaches to help slow down negative thinking.

Brief Introduction to Stress Hormones

The body creates cortisol when you feel under stress. This hormone makes your heart beat faster and your senses more alert. It can be helpful for short-term dangers, but with heartbreak, there is often no quick fix. Prolonged stress can wear down the body. That is why managing stress is an important part of healing.

Surprising Methods That Can Help

1. **Laughing on Purpose**: Even fake laughter can help reduce stress. There are laughter therapy groups where people gather to laugh for no reason. The body responds to the act of laughing, releasing endorphins.
2. **Singing**: Singing, even if you are not good at it, can help regulate breathing and improve mood. It can be done at home, in your car, or anywhere you feel comfortable.

The Balance of Emotions and Logic

Some people try to rely only on logic and ignore their feelings. Others swim in their emotions and forget logic. Healing from heartbreak requires both sides. You can feel sad while still making practical plans. You can acknowledge anger while choosing not to lash out in destructive ways.

Why Emotional Intelligence Matters

Emotional intelligence is the skill of recognizing your own emotions and those of others. It also involves managing your emotions in a healthy way. After heartbreak, boosting your emotional intelligence can help you respond better to stress, communicate more effectively, and avoid repeating harmful relationship patterns in the future.

Conclusion of Chapter 2

The emotional effects of heartbreak can be large, and they can show up in many aspects of your life. You might feel sadness, anger, or confusion. Your mind might get stuck on negative thoughts. Remember, these reactions are normal for a situation involving loss. The mind can respond as if you are in physical danger, releasing stress hormones and triggering strong emotions.

But there are ways to help ease these reactions: limit rumination, find small physical activities, and manage your thoughts with real coping strategies. By learning how heartbreak affects your mind, you can gain more control over your feelings and start to move forward in a healthier way.

In the next chapters, we will cover the physical impact of sadness on the body, common mistakes people make after a breakup, and more detailed ways to handle the different stages of heartbreak. This will help you see the full picture of how heartbreak touches every part of a person's life—and what to do to become stronger step by step.

Chapter 3: Physical Effects of Sadness

After a breakup, sadness is not just an emotional experience. It can affect the body in powerful ways. Many people do not realize that heartbreak can create real physical symptoms. This chapter will explain some of the common and less common ways sadness can appear in the body. We will also look at methods to manage these effects. Understanding these signs can help you see that you are not simply "weak" or "lazy." Instead, your body is adjusting to a major emotional loss.

Common Physical Reactions

1. **Changes in Appetite**
    - **Loss of Appetite**: Some women find it hard to eat after heartbreak. They feel a tightness in the stomach, or they simply do not feel hungry. If this goes on for too long, it can lead to weight loss, fatigue, and nutrient deficiencies.
    - **Increased Appetite**: Others might eat more than usual, especially sugary or fatty foods. This can be a quick way to feel comfort. However, overeating can lead to weight gain, sluggishness, and guilt.
2. **Trouble Sleeping**
    - **Insomnia**: Many women have trouble falling asleep or staying asleep when they are sad. The mind can replay events, making the brain too active at bedtime.
    - **Excessive Sleeping**: On the flip side, some may sleep a lot to escape the pain. While rest is good, too much sleep can lead to low energy and a feeling of disconnection from daily life.
3. **Headaches and Body Aches**
    - **Tension Headaches**: Stress can cause muscles in the neck and scalp to tighten, leading to headaches that feel like a band around the head.
    - **Stomach Pains**: The gut is sensitive to emotional changes. Heartbreak can bring stomach cramps or digestion issues.
    - **General Aches**: Some people experience random aches or pains in their body. These might appear in the shoulders, back, or chest region due to muscle tension.
4. **Energy Fluctuations**

- **Fatigue**: Feeling emotionally drained can translate to physical fatigue. Even simple tasks might feel overwhelming.
- **Restlessness**: Others may experience an inability to sit still. They might pace around, feeling a surge of nervous energy from stress hormones.

Why Emotional Pain Feels Physical

Research shows that the brain does not neatly separate emotional and physical pain. When a person is in deep emotional distress, areas of the brain responsible for sensing physical pain can become active. This overlap means that heartbreak can feel like a true pain in the chest or gut, even though there is no direct physical injury.

Stress Hormones: During heartbreak, stress hormones like cortisol and adrenaline can flood your system. Cortisol can affect metabolism, sleep, and even immune function. Too much cortisol for a long time can weaken the body, making you more prone to illness.

Lesser-Known Physical Responses

1. **Skin Problems**
   - Sometimes heartbreak can trigger acne flare-ups or rashes due to the stress response. The skin is an organ that can react to emotional strain in surprising ways.
2. **Teeth Grinding**
   - Women under emotional pressure might grind their teeth at night or clench their jaw during the day. This can lead to jaw pain, headaches, and dental issues if it continues.
3. **Hair Changes**
   - In very stressful cases, some individuals report hair shedding. This does not happen to everyone, but it can occur if the body remains in a stressed state for a long period.
4. **Hormonal Imbalances**
   - Stress can disrupt normal hormone levels, affecting things like the menstrual cycle or thyroid function. It is worth noting that not everyone experiences these changes, but it is possible for heartbreak stress to spill over into hormonal health.

Managing Physical Effects

1. **Nutrition Tips**
   - **Gentle Meals**: If you are not hungry, try small meals or nutritious liquids like broth-based soups or smoothies. This can help you get vitamins and minerals without forcing a heavy meal.
   - **Balanced Choices**: If you are overeating, keep easy and healthy foods on hand: fruits, nuts, or whole-grain snacks. This reduces the chance of reaching for junk food.
2. **Sleep Hygiene**
   - **Set a Bedtime**: Going to sleep at the same time each night can help train your body to rest.
   - **No Screens Before Bed**: The light from phones or tablets can trick your brain into staying awake. Try to stop screen use at least 30 minutes before bedtime.
   - **Calming Rituals**: A warm shower or soft music can signal to your body that it's time to relax.
3. **Physical Exercise**
   - **Low-Impact Routines**: If you feel very tired, gentle stretching or a slow walk can help. You do not need to do a heavy workout.
   - **Short Bursts**: If you are restless, a quick burst of exercise—like jumping jacks or dancing to a favorite song—can help burn off some nervous energy.
   - **Nature Walks**: Spending time in natural settings can calm the mind and soothe the body. Studies suggest that being around greenery can help lower stress levels.
4. **Soothing the Muscles**
   - **Warm Baths**: Heat can relax tight muscles. Adding simple bath salts might help ease tension.
   - **Massage or Self-Massage**: You can press gently on your shoulders or neck to release knots of tension.
   - **Progressive Muscle Relaxation**: Tense and then release different muscle groups, starting from the feet up to the head. This can reduce stress signals in the body.

Uncommon Insights for Physical Self-Care

- **Foot Soaks with Epsom Salt**: This simple practice can help relax not only the feet but also the mind. The magnesium in Epsom salts can help calm the nervous system.

- **Aromatherapy**: Certain scents like lavender or chamomile may assist in lowering stress. Placing a drop on your pillow or using a diffuser can create a calming environment.
- **Simple Acupressure**: Pressing on the space between the thumb and index finger can help relieve tension headaches. You can also press on the area above the nose bridge between the eyebrows to reduce stress.

Keeping Medical Checkups in Mind

When sadness lingers, it can weaken your immune system. If you notice you are catching colds more often or feeling physically unwell for long stretches, it might be wise to see a healthcare professional. A doctor can check if there are any underlying issues that might be worsened by stress. They can also give advice on vitamins or supplements to support your body during emotional distress.

Red Flags to Watch Out For

- **Continual Weight Loss or Gain**: If your weight is changing rapidly, it is worth monitoring more closely.
- **Chest Pain**: Always get chest pain checked out, even if you suspect it is from heartbreak. Real heart issues can sometimes blend with emotional stress.
- **Constant Exhaustion**: Feeling tired all day, every day, for weeks might point to a deeper issue, like depression or thyroid problems.
- **Frequent Illness**: If you are getting sick more often than usual, it might be a sign that your body is under too much stress.

Tying Emotional and Physical Care Together

Caring for your body can help care for your mind, and caring for your mind can help your body. They are connected. If you ignore your physical needs, emotional progress might be slower. If you ignore your emotional wounds, your body might keep sounding the alarm through aches, insomnia, or other issues.

A few ways to integrate both:

- **Mindful Breathing**: Spend a minute or two each day focusing on your breath. Inhale slowly through your nose, hold for a short count, and exhale through your mouth. This helps calm the nervous system.

- **Writing Down Symptoms**: Keep a short journal of how you feel physically. Note if there is any pattern tied to your emotions. You might see that certain triggers cause headaches or stomach discomfort.
- **Check Your Posture**: Heartbreak can lead to slouching or curling into yourself when you feel defeated. Straighten your spine, roll your shoulders back, and take a deep breath. This posture shift can boost mood and energy.

Strategies for Work and School

If you have obligations like work or classes, physical sadness can interfere with your performance. Here are some steps to cope:

1. **Plan Small Breaks**: Stand up, stretch, or walk a little every hour. This helps reduce tension in the body.
2. **Stay Hydrated**: Drinking enough water is a simple way to keep your body functioning well. Dehydration can worsen fatigue and headaches.
3. **Pack Healthy Snacks**: To avoid reaching for sugary treats when stress spikes, keep balanced snacks at your desk or in your bag.
4. **Speak Up When Needed**: If you have a supportive boss or teacher, let them know you are going through a rough time. You do not have to share details, but a quick note that you are under stress might help them understand if you need flexibility.

Creating a Gentle Routine

A routine can bring structure when you feel lost:

- **Morning Ritual**: Wake up at the same time, drink a glass of water, and do a brief stretch or writing exercise.
- **Mid-Day Pause**: Take 5-10 minutes after lunch to breathe quietly or walk.
- **Evening Wind-Down**: One hour before bed, lower the lights and do a calm activity like reading a simple book or listening to gentle sounds.

The Role of Relaxation Practices

- **Guided Muscle Relaxation**: Lie down, close your eyes, and focus on each muscle group. Tense each group for 5 seconds, then release. Move from your toes to your forehead.
- **Light Stretching**: Gentle stretching at night can help calm tight muscles.

- **Non-Distracting Activities**: Activities like painting, knitting, or simple puzzles can calm the mind. They do not require deep analysis, giving your mind a break from heartbreak thoughts.

Handling Social Media and Physical Health Together

Social media can influence how you feel about your body and your healing process. Seeing posts about others who seem happy can affect your mood. This stress can worsen physical symptoms. Setting time limits for social media or muting certain accounts might reduce added pressure on your mind and body. A calmer mind often means a calmer body.

Realistic Expectations for Recovery

Recovery from heartbreak is not a quick fix. Physical symptoms usually improve as your emotional state stabilizes. Some days you might feel strong, and other days you might feel weak. It is normal to fluctuate. By staying aware of your physical health, you give yourself the best chance to heal fully.

Special Note on Self-Harm or Destructive Patterns

A small number of people might turn to self-harm, such as cutting or burning themselves, when they feel overwhelming sadness. If you find yourself thinking of harming your body in any way, please seek help immediately from a mental health professional or a trusted support line. There is no shame in asking for help.

Concluding Thoughts for Chapter 3

The body and mind work together during heartbreak. It is important to remember that physical symptoms of sadness are genuine responses. This is not a sign of being overly dramatic or unable to handle life. It is a sign that your body is under a form of stress that needs care and attention.

Moving forward, keep track of what your body is telling you. Adjust your eating, sleeping, and activity patterns in gentle ways. By addressing physical needs, you also support your emotional healing. In the next chapter, we will examine common mistakes that people make after a breakup. Understanding these pitfalls can help you avoid prolonging your heartbreak. Being mindful of both your emotional and physical well-being will serve as a foundation for healthier days ahead.

Chapter 4: Common Mistakes People Make After a Breakup

When a relationship ends, it is normal to feel disoriented. Emotions run high, and it is easy to make choices that do more harm than good. This chapter looks at the most common mistakes people make after a breakup, including ones that might feel useful in the moment but lead to problems later on. We will discuss each mistake in detail and explore better alternatives.

1. Rushing into a New Relationship

A quick rebound is one of the most frequent errors made after heartbreak. People can be tempted to fill the void by dating someone else right away. While it may give temporary comfort, it rarely addresses the root problems.

- **Why This Happens**: Loneliness can be intense, and attention from a new person can distract from sadness. Some individuals also seek revenge or validation by showing they have "moved on."
- **Long-Term Effects**: If the issues from the past relationship are not resolved, they often resurface. Emotional baggage can carry into the new relationship, creating a cycle of unhealthy connections.
- **Healthier Choice**: Allow some time to reflect on what went wrong and what you need. It is helpful to find a stable emotional footing before entering another relationship.

2. Staying in Constant Contact with the Ex

Another common mistake is trying to maintain frequent contact with the ex-partner out of a fear of losing them fully. Some people believe remaining "friends" right away will soften the blow.

- **Why This Happens**: Hope that the relationship might restart. Also, the fear of completely losing a person who once played a significant role in life.
- **Problems That Can Arise**: Continuous communication can reopen wounds and delay recovery. You may misinterpret friendly gestures as romantic interest and stay stuck in emotional turmoil.

- **Better Approach**: A period of little to no contact can give both sides space to heal. If a friendship is possible later, it usually works better when both parties have moved on emotionally.

3. Using Substances to Numb the Pain

Some individuals turn to alcohol, drugs, or excessive partying to block out the pain of heartbreak.

- **Immediate Effect**: Substances can temporarily mask sadness or anxiety.
- **Long-Term Consequences**: Dependence can form, leading to further emotional and physical harm. Overuse of substances can also create financial problems and damage other relationships.
- **Wiser Alternative**: Seek healthier outlets like physical activities, creative pursuits, or talking to supportive friends. If you feel you are leaning on substances too often, consider speaking to a counselor.

4. Public Venting or Oversharing on Social Media

In the age of online platforms, many go online to share every feeling. They might post long emotional updates about their heartbreak or throw passive-aggressive comments at the ex.

- **Why People Do It**: Looking for sympathy, wanting to shame the ex, or craving a sense of release.
- **Downside**: Public posts can attract unwanted attention, judgement, and even more drama. Negative or personal details about the relationship can also remain on the internet for a long time.
- **Smarter Path**: Express your feelings in a private journal or in face-to-face talks with friends. This method respects both your privacy and emotional well-being.

5. Blaming Everything on the Ex or Yourself

Blame is an easy trap. Some blame their ex completely, while others place all the blame on themselves.

- **When You Blame the Ex Fully**: You risk not seeing your own part in the relationship issues. This can make you repeat patterns with new partners.

- **When You Blame Yourself Entirely**: You might sink into guilt and shame, lowering your confidence. This can lead to fear of connecting with someone again.
- **Balanced View**: Few breakups happen without some level of shared responsibility. It is more productive to look at the relationship as a whole, acknowledge mistakes from both sides, and learn from them.

6. Isolating from Support Systems

Some people feel so hurt that they withdraw from friends, family, or social events. They stop picking up calls and lose touch with the outside world.

- **Why This Feels Comforting**: Isolation can feel like a protective shell. You might think you are sparing others from your sadness or that you cannot handle any social interaction.
- **Negative Effects**: Lack of social contact can worsen loneliness and sadness. It can also prolong negative thinking if you have no one to talk to.
- **Healthier Method**: Seek out at least one or two trusted individuals. Even if you do not want large gatherings, having a small circle of support can make a huge difference.

7. Seeking Revenge

Anger can lead people to do harmful things to "get back" at the ex, such as spreading rumors, damaging property, or trying to turn mutual friends against the person.

- **Immediate Satisfaction**: Revenge might bring a temporary rush of power, but it rarely fixes emotional pain.
- **Long-Lasting Problems**: You might regret these actions later, and they could harm your reputation or lead to legal trouble.
- **Positive Alternative**: Channel anger into something useful, like physical exercise or finishing a personal project. Focus on rebuilding your own life rather than tearing down someone else's.

8. Clinging to Idealized Memories

Heartbreak can distort memories. You might only remember the good times, forgetting the arguments or the reasons for the breakup.

- **Why This Happens**: Emotional longing can make the past seem better than it was. This romanticized view keeps hope alive, even when the relationship was flawed.
- **Danger of This Mindset**: You might try to return to a relationship that was unhealthy or keep yourself from moving forward.
- **Grounding Exercise**: Write down specific problems in the relationship. This helps you see the reality more clearly and avoid glossing over negatives.

9. Letting Physical Health Slip

As mentioned in the previous chapter, heartbreak can drain energy. Many neglect exercise, meals, or hygiene.

- **Root Cause**: Depression-like symptoms or pure lack of motivation might lead to ignoring health.
- **Snowball Effect**: Poor health habits can worsen mood, creating a cycle of feeling worse physically and emotionally.
- **Step-by-Step Fix**: Focus on small improvements—like adding a daily walk or making one healthy meal a day—to gradually return to better self-care.

10. Bottling Up Feelings

Some people refuse to cry or talk about the breakup because they want to appear strong or they think acknowledging sadness makes it worse.

- **Immediate Seeming Benefit**: You might feel you are keeping control by suppressing tears or anger.
- **Long-Term Risk**: Emotions kept inside can lead to bigger breakdowns later or can morph into stress-related health problems.
- **Healthy Release**: Choose a private setting or a trusted friend to share emotions. Writing them down can also be a safe outlet.

Uncommon Mistakes That People Rarely Discuss

1. **Forcing a Friendship Right Away**
   - While it is fine to maintain a respectful connection someday, pushing a friendship too early can create confusion. You might be drawn into emotional conflicts or jealousy, preventing both of you from healing properly.
2. **Seeking Closure in the Wrong Places**

- Many look for closure in repeated talks with the ex, hoping for a clear explanation or apology. Sometimes closure never comes in the way you expect. Relying on your ex to heal your heartbreak may keep you stuck.

3. **Ignoring Red Flags from Your Own Behavior**
    - After heartbreak, you might see patterns in how you approach love or handle conflicts. Ignoring these insights can lead you to repeat them in the next relationship. Being aware of your own tendencies can help you break unhealthy cycles.
4. **Trying to Fix the Ex's Life**
    - Some people offer themselves as a "helper" to their ex, believing this will keep them close. This often leads to more pain if the ex takes advantage of this help or if it stirs new arguments.
5. **Making Impulsive Financial Decisions**
    - Emotional distress can cloud judgment. People might buy expensive items or give money to their ex out of guilt or an attempt to hold onto the connection. This can lead to regrettable financial strain.

Why We Fall into These Mistakes

When the heart is hurting, it becomes difficult to see things clearly. The brain is in a heightened emotional state, and the drive to reduce pain can lead to reckless or poorly thought-out actions. Also, we might seek to restore control in our lives by doing something dramatic or seeking attention from the ex or from others.

Better Ways to Handle Post-Breakup Traps

- **Pause and Reflect**: Before acting on a strong emotion, take a moment. Count to ten, take a few slow breaths, or step out of the room. Even a short pause can prevent a knee-jerk mistake.
- **Focus on Self-Improvement**: Put energy into activities or goals that build you up, such as learning a new skill, reading books, or engaging in small home projects. This approach redirects your mind from the breakup and towards personal growth.
- **Talk It Out**: Conversations with supportive people can give you a reality check. They might point out how your actions could harm you in the long run. Friends and family often see patterns you may overlook.

- **Seek Professional Guidance**: Therapists or counselors are trained to help people navigate breakups. They can give a neutral perspective and tools for dealing with emotional pain.

The Value of Setting Boundaries

Setting boundaries protects your emotional health. These include:

1. **Limiting Communication with the Ex**: Decide on the type and frequency of contact. In many cases, zero contact for a period of time is beneficial.
2. **Social Media Boundaries**: If you find yourself stalking the ex's profile or feeling hurt by their posts, consider muting or blocking them.
3. **Time Boundaries with Others**: It is okay to let friends know that certain topics are off-limits if you are not ready to talk about them.

Personal Examples to Illustrate Common Mistakes (Fictional but Realistic)

1. **Rushing into Rebound**
    - **Anna** ended a two-year relationship and jumped into dating within a week. She felt good for a short time, but found that her emotions were still tied to her ex. Her new partner became confused by her mixed signals, leading to another painful split.
2. **Oversharing on Social Media**
    - **Bella** wrote daily posts about her heartbreak, blaming her ex in detailed posts. She found that old mutual friends started avoiding her, and her boss at work expressed concern about her emotional well-being. Bella realized this method backfired, creating more tension in her life.
3. **Seeking Closure Through Endless Calls**
    - **Chloe** kept calling her ex, looking for answers about why the relationship ended. She felt each call made her more upset. The ex gave vague reasons, and the repeated contact only stirred more confusion.

Specific Tips to Avoid Common Pitfalls

- **Plan for Lonely Moments**: Loneliness often leads to calls or messages you might regret. Write down a list of other activities you can do when the urge hits: watch a comedy, take a walk, or call a friend.

- **Remove Tempting Reminders**: If certain gifts or photos trigger urges to contact your ex, store them out of sight. This physical change can help you emotionally.
- **Give Yourself 30 Days**: Some people find it helpful to commit to no contact for at least 30 days. This gives the mind time to settle before deciding on any relationship with the ex.
- **Constructive Anger Release**: If you feel the desire for revenge, channel that anger into something useful, like working out or cleaning your space. Physical tasks can help burn off angry energy in a safer way.

How to Step Back from a Mistake Already Made

We are not perfect. Sometimes we realize too late that we have acted in a way that is not helpful.

- **Accept It and Move On**: It does not define you. Acknowledge the mistake and focus on what you learned.
- **Correct It If Possible**: If you posted something hurtful about your ex, consider removing it or posting a brief apology if it caused harm.
- **Set New Boundaries**: If the mistake involved contact or self-destructive behavior, decide on a new plan to prevent a repeat. That might mean blocking numbers or committing to counseling.

The Importance of Forgiving Yourself

Sometimes heartbreak can lead to shame, especially if you feel you "failed" in the relationship. Or if you made mistakes like sending angry texts or calling your ex's workplace. Remember, you are human. Give yourself room to learn from these actions. Holding onto self-blame can keep you in a negative place.

Building a Supportive Environment

- **Identify Supportive People**: Not everyone will understand your pain. Choose those who listen without judging or pushing their own agendas.
- **Consider a Support Group**: Local or online groups exist for people going through breakups. Sharing experiences with others in the same situation can give relief and insights.
- **Limit Time with Negative Influences**: If certain friends urge you to do unwise things, take a temporary break from them to keep yourself stable.

Final Words on Avoiding Common Mistakes

Everyone handles heartbreak differently. There is no single "correct" way to heal. However, avoiding these common mistakes can make the process smoother. You will likely still feel sadness, anger, or frustration, but you can spare yourself extra complications by stepping back before taking rash actions.

Key Reminders:

- Quick fixes often lead to long-term issues.
- Boundaries with an ex and with yourself are crucial.
- Lean on supportive friends or professionals.
- Learn from the breakup so you do not repeat old patterns.

In the next chapters, we will look at healthy ways to let out deep sadness, handle loss of self-worth, and more. Knowing what *not* to do is a big step, but you also need to fill that gap with constructive actions and self-care methods. By steering clear of these pitfalls, you give yourself a clearer path to actual healing.

Chapter 5: Healthy Ways to Express Sad Feelings

Sadness can sometimes feel like a heavy load that weighs you down. After heartbreak, many women struggle with how to let this emotion out. Some try to hold it in, worried that showing sadness means weakness. Others might let it explode in anger or tears that feel uncontrollable. In this chapter, we will look at many healthy ways to let out sadness. We will discuss strategies that let you express deep emotions without harming yourself or others. We will also look at lesser-known methods that can help you process your feelings in a more balanced way.

Why Expressing Sadness Matters

When sadness is not released, it can build up like pressure in a closed container. This can turn into anxiety, physical pain, or a sense of numbness. Expressing sadness in a healthy manner does not make you a weak person. In fact, it can help you heal faster and protect you from bigger emotional distress in the future.

- **Maintaining Emotional Health**: Releasing sadness can help you avoid feeling stuck. It provides a channel for strong emotions, giving them a place to go instead of lingering in your mind.
- **Promoting Honesty**: When you express your sadness, you are admitting to yourself and others that something hurts. Honesty can lead to clarity about what you need to feel better.
- **Preventing Emotional Outbursts**: Bottled-up sadness can cause random meltdowns or bursts of anger. Healthy expression helps prevent these surprises.

The Risk of Bottling Up Emotions

Many women fear that if they start crying, they will never stop. Or they worry friends might see them as unstable if they openly share their grief. These fears can lead to a habit of hiding pain behind a mask of "I'm fine."

- **Emotional Overflow**: When you do not release sadness, it can come out in unwanted ways later. You might find yourself crying at work over something small or snapping at a friend for no real reason.
- **Physical Tension**: Suppressed emotions can cause muscle tightness, headaches, or even digestive problems. This happens because the mind and body are connected.
- **Higher Stress**: Keeping sadness locked away can raise levels of stress hormones in the body. Over time, this can affect your health, weaken your immune system, and make you feel constantly on edge.

Different Avenues for Expression

You do not have to follow just one method to express sadness. It is often helpful to mix several approaches, finding the right balance for you. Below are various channels you can use:

1. **Art-Based Expression**
    - **Painting or Drawing**: Some people find it easier to communicate feelings through colors and shapes instead of words. You do not need to be a great artist to paint or sketch what you feel.
    - **Sculpting with Clay**: Working with your hands can be calming. The act of molding clay or any similar material can help you release tension and keep you focused on creating something.
    - **Collage Making**: Collect magazines or images that represent different emotions. Cutting and pasting these together can help you see your sadness from a new angle.
2. **Physical-Based Expression**
    - **Dance or Movement**: Turning on music and allowing your body to move freely can release stored tension. You do not need fancy steps—just let the music guide your movements.
    - **Mindful Stretching**: Slow, gentle stretches can help you become aware of where sadness sits in your body. You can focus on releasing tension in your shoulders, back, or hips.
    - **Drumming or Tapping**: Some people find relief by tapping rhythms on a drum or even on a table. Repetitive tapping can match the beat of your heart and help you feel connected to the present moment.
3. **Verbal Expression**

- **Talking to a Friend**: Choose someone you trust who will listen without judging or rushing you. Speaking your sadness out loud can make it feel less heavy.
- **Voice Recording**: If you are uncomfortable talking face to face, try recording yourself on your phone. You can speak freely about your pain, then listen back to understand your emotional patterns.
- **Therapy Sessions**: Professional counselors are trained to help you deal with heartbreak. They provide a safe space to express sadness and can offer useful perspectives on your situation.

4. **Written Expression**
   - **Detailed Journaling**: Dedicate a notebook to writing exactly how you feel each day. You can detail your thoughts, frustrations, and hopes. It is a private outlet that is always available.
   - **Poetry or Short Stories**: Even simple poems can capture big feelings. Fictional stories let you indirectly explore your heartbreak by using characters and plots.
   - **Letters**: Write a letter to your ex-partner or to yourself. You do not have to send it. This method often brings clarity to mixed emotions.

5. **Nature-Inspired Expression**
   - **Walking in Green Spaces**: Nature can calm the mind. Talking out loud while walking alone in a park can help you let out sadness.
   - **Gardening**: Tending to plants can bring a sense of peace. You can bury notes in the soil as a symbolic way of releasing pain.
   - **Sky Gazing**: Simply lying down and looking up at the clouds can create a sense of perspective. It might help you feel less overwhelmed.

Setting a Safe Environment for Emotional Release

It is important to find or create a space where you feel secure. Some people cry more easily in the shower, where the sound of running water masks tears. Others prefer a quiet room with soft lighting. Here are some tips:

- **Choose a Time and Place**: If you live with others, pick a time when you will not be disturbed. Turn off your phone to avoid distractions.
- **Gather Comfort Items**: A blanket, tissues, or even a stuffed toy can provide a sense of safety.

- **Have a Calming Activity Ready**: After you release sadness, you might feel raw. It can help to have a simple activity, like a coloring book or gentle music, to ease yourself back to a stable state.

Singing or Humming as an Emotional Outlet

One approach that people often overlook is singing or humming. You do not have to sing well to gain the benefits:

- **Regulates Breathing**: Singing forces you to take deeper breaths, which can calm your nerves.
- **Releases Energy**: Belt out a sad song or a slow tune. This can be a powerful way to free emotions locked inside.
- **Personal Concerts**: If you are shy, sing in your car or when you are alone at home.

Out-of-the-Ordinary Methods

Sometimes simple suggestions do not fully resonate. Below are some lesser-known ways to express sadness:

1. **Writing Sadness on Paper, Then Shredding It**
   - Jot down every painful thought. Use strong words if needed. Afterward, tear the paper into small pieces or shred it. This act can feel like a release.
2. **Clay Smash**
   - Take a piece of clay or dough and form it into an object that represents your sadness or heartbreak. Then, smash it gently. Watching it lose shape can be a symbolic way to show that pain can change form and eventually dissolve.
3. **Scream Therapy**
   - In some places, people gather to scream into the air or into pillows. This might sound odd, but letting out a good shout in a safe space (like in your car or into a cushion at home) can lift tension from your body.
4. **Painting With Water on a Wall or Pavement**

- Using just water and a brush, paint strokes on a sidewalk or wall. Watch as they disappear. This can represent the passing of sadness over time.

Maintaining a Balance: Not Overdoing Expression

While it is healthy to let sadness out, some people might stay in a constant state of sadness expression. They cry daily for months without seeking ways to move forward. Here are some reminders:

- **Set Time Limits**: If you choose to write or paint about your sadness, consider giving yourself a certain amount of time each day for that activity.
- **Alternate with Positive Action**: After you express sadness, do something kind for yourself. That might be reading an uplifting story, watching a funny show, or talking to a friend about a lighter topic.

Coping with Criticism from Others

Some family members or friends might say things like, "Stop whining," or "You should be over it by now." This can make you feel guilty about expressing sadness. However, healing is not a race.

- **Communicate Your Needs**: Calmly explain that you need time and safe ways to let out your emotions.
- **Distance If Necessary**: If certain people continue to dismiss or mock your feelings, it might help to limit contact until you are stronger emotionally.
- **Find Empathetic Allies**: Seek out friends, online forums, or support groups where people understand heartbreak. Their feedback can encourage you to keep healing.

Pairing Expression with Self-Soothing Techniques

After letting out sadness, you might feel empty or exhausted. Self-soothing can fill that gap:

- **Warm Shower or Bath**: Let the water relax your muscles and wash away physical tension.
- **Cozy Clothing**: Slip into something soft, like warm socks or a comfortable sweater.
- **Light Aromatic Candles**: Use mild scents like vanilla or mild citrus. Strong smells can sometimes irritate the senses after an emotional release.
- **Gentle Self-Massage**: Rub your shoulders, neck, and hands. This can calm your nervous system.

Helping Children or Dependents Understand

If you are a mother or caregiver, children might see you expressing sadness. They may ask questions or even feel worried.

- **Age-Appropriate Explanations**: You can say, "I am sad because something hurt my feelings," and reassure them that sadness is normal and will pass.
- **Show Healthy Expression**: Let them see that it is okay to cry or talk about pain in a calm way. This can teach them good emotional habits.
- **Ask for Help**: If you have supportive family or friends, let them babysit for a few hours so you can have private time to express sadness.

Group Activities for Expression

Sometimes sharing sadness with others going through a similar heartbreak can be healing. Group settings can offer comfort, but be mindful of picking the right group.

- **Support Circles**: These are often led by a counselor or a trained leader. Members share stories and encourage each other.
- **Art Therapy Workshops**: These workshops guide participants in art projects that help process various emotions.
- **Movement Sessions**: Some communities offer group dance classes designed for emotional release. The collective movement can foster a sense of unity.

Digital Avenues of Expression

If you cannot attend in-person sessions, online resources might help:

- **Anonymous Forums**: Places on the internet where you can post your thoughts without revealing your real name. This can be a good release when you feel isolated.
- **Video Diaries**: Record short clips of yourself speaking about your daily emotional state. Store them privately or share with a counselor if you choose.
- **Creative Apps**: Some apps allow for doodling, painting, or creating music. These can be quick outlets for sadness on the go.

Gauging Your Progress

You might wonder if your sadness expression is making a difference. Here are signs that you are moving forward in a healthy way:

- **More Emotional Clarity**: Over time, you will notice you can name your emotions more easily. Instead of just feeling overwhelmed, you might identify a sense of longing, anger, or regret.
- **Less Sudden Overwhelm**: You begin to have fewer random outbursts. When sadness arrives, you have tools to deal with it.
- **Better Sleep or Appetite**: Healthy expression can improve physical issues like insomnia or poor eating habits.
- **Moments of Calm**: Even if you still feel waves of sadness, you might also feel calmer or lighter in between those waves.

Handling Guilt or Shame

Sometimes, heartbreak carries guilt. You might feel responsible for the breakup or think you did not handle the relationship well. Expressing sadness might also bring guilt if you were taught that emotional display is bad.

- **Self-Compassion**: Speak kindly to yourself. Remind yourself that mistakes happen, and heartbreak does not mean you are a bad person.

- **Rewrite Your Inner Script**: Instead of "I should be ashamed," try, "I am learning from a hard experience."
- **Seek Professional Input**: If guilt becomes overwhelming, a counselor can guide you toward forgiving yourself and moving on.

The Role of Gratitude

Although this chapter is about expressing sadness, finding small things to appreciate can balance deep grief. For instance, after a good cry, you might spend a moment thinking about one positive aspect of your life—a loyal friend, a comfortable home, or a skill you possess. This does not erase sadness, but it keeps a window open for other feelings as well.

Combining Expression with Goals

When sadness is shared in a healthy manner, you free your mind to focus on other parts of life. It can help to pair your emotional expression with small daily goals:

- **Tiny Steps**: After journaling in the morning, list one thing you want to do that day (like preparing a simple meal or organizing a corner of your room).
- **Positive Affirmations**: Use short statements: "I handled my sadness today, and that is progress."
- **Track Milestones**: You might write down that you cried less frequently this week or you talked openly with a friend about your heartbreak. Recognizing these milestones can motivate you to keep going.

Surprising Tips for Emotional Expression

- **Melted Wax Drawing**: Melt old crayons or candle wax and pour them on a sheet of paper to create abstract shapes. It can be a visual representation of how your sadness flows out.

- **Sound Bath at Home**: You can create relaxing tones using singing bowls or even online sound therapy clips. Lying quietly while these sounds play can gently release pent-up feelings.
- **Picture Tearing**: If you have photos that bring you heartache, you can tear them up. You could also store them away if tearing them feels too extreme. Either action can help you control the memories you see daily.

Finding What Works for You

Not every form of expression will fit your style. Some might find it silly to dance alone or record voice notes. Others might find journaling too tedious. Feel free to try different methods and see what feels right. The goal is not to add more pressure to your life; it is to relieve it.

- **Test Before Dismissing**: Give each method a fair try. Sometimes it takes a few attempts to feel comfortable.
- **Combine Methods**: For example, you could journal in the morning, paint in the afternoon, and talk to a friend at night.
- **Trust Your Instincts**: If a method is making you feel worse or too exposed, it may not be right for you at that moment.

Conclusion of Chapter 5

Expressing sadness is an important part of healing from heartbreak. Rather than letting sorrow build up, you can channel it through art, writing, movement, verbal expression, or nature-based activities. Finding a safe environment and a helpful technique can reduce the emotional strain you are carrying. When sadness has a place to go, you are less likely to feel overwhelmed or stuck.

As you experiment with different methods, stay mindful of how your body and mind react. Notice small improvements in your mood or clarity. In the next chapter, we will look at the loss of self-worth that often follows heartbreak. We will talk about why it happens and how to rebuild a healthier sense of self so you can stand firm in your value and potential.

Chapter 6: Dealing with Loss of Self-Worth

Breakups can leave a lasting mark on how you see yourself. Many women say they feel "not good enough" after a relationship ends. They might think they caused the failure or that they are no longer lovable. This chapter will dive into the concept of self-worth, why it takes a hit during heartbreak, and how to rebuild it step by step. Feeling valuable is not about being perfect. It is about recognizing that you have qualities worth respecting, no matter what happened in your past.

Why Does Self-Worth Plummet After Heartbreak?

When you share your life with someone, you often share your dreams, secrets, and vulnerabilities. After a breakup, you might feel that the trust you gave was wasted or that you were a "bad partner." Even if the split was not your fault, doubts can crawl into your mind. You may question whether you are attractive enough, smart enough, or kind enough to keep someone's love.

- **Personal Investment**: Romantic ties usually involve deep emotional and psychological investment. When it ends, you might believe you lost a part of yourself.
- **Social Judgments**: Friends or family might ask insensitive questions like, "Why did it fail?" or "What did you do wrong?" These remarks can make you blame yourself.
- **Cultural Pressure**: Some societies put a lot of weight on being in a partnership. If a relationship ends, a woman might feel she has broken some unwritten rule.

Common Signs of Low Self-Worth

1. **Negative Self-Talk**: You catch yourself frequently thinking, "I'm useless," or "I never get anything right."
2. **Seeking Constant Approval**: You look to others to tell you that you are okay, pretty, or capable. You might fear making decisions alone.
3. **Fear of Trying New Things**: You do not apply for a new job, take on a new hobby, or go to new places because you do not believe you can succeed.

4. **People-Pleasing**: You might bend over backwards to make others happy, fearing rejection if you say "no."
5. **Comparisons**: You compare yourself to your ex's new partner or to people on social media, always finding yourself lacking.

How Heartbreak Magnifies These Feelings

When heartbreak enters the picture, it acts like a magnifying glass. Small insecurities become huge. You might remember every mistake you made in the relationship and convince yourself these flaws led to the end. Meanwhile, you might overlook the good things you did.

- **Logical Errors**: Emotionally, you might jump to conclusions: "They left me, so I must be worthless." But one event does not define your entire worth.
- **Memory Distortions**: You might forget the times your partner praised you, focusing only on criticisms or arguments.
- **Comparison with Others**: If your ex moves on quickly, you might imagine that the new partner is better than you in every way.

First Steps to Regain Self-Worth

1. **Acknowledge the Gap**: Understand that heartbreak has impacted how you see yourself. Recognize that these negative thoughts might not be factual.
2. **Identify Your Strengths**: List qualities you appreciate about yourself, such as kindness, empathy, or a good sense of humor. They do not have to be huge traits. Even small positive traits matter.
3. **Stay Aware of Negativity**: Each time a harmful thought like, "I'm worthless," appears, pause and label it. Telling yourself, "This is just a negative thought" can lessen its grip.

Building Self-Worth Day by Day

1. Small Achievements

- **Set Mini-Goals**: Aim for goals you know you can reach, like reading a few pages of a book each day or learning a short cooking recipe.
- **Track Progress**: Write down what you have achieved daily. Seeing it on paper can remind you that you are capable of growth.

2. Positive Self-Talk

- **Use Affirmations**: Short phrases like "I am capable," or "I deserve respect" said daily can create a new internal script.
- **Rephrase Errors**: When you make a mistake, say, "I made a mistake," instead of "I am a failure."

3. Healthy Social Circles

- **Supportive People Only**: Spend time with friends who value you. Limit time with those who constantly criticize or belittle you.
- **Honest Communication**: If a friend or family member says something hurtful, calmly let them know how it affects you. This sets boundaries that protect your self-worth.

Recognizing Outside Influences on Your Self-Worth

Sometimes, heartbreak can stir up old wounds from childhood. For instance, if you grew up feeling you had to earn love by being perfect, a breakup might confirm that fear. If you had a parent who was emotionally distant, you might feel unworthy of love when a partner leaves.

- **Possible Past Triggers**:
    - Parents who rarely gave praise
    - Bullying experiences at school
    - Past failed relationships
- **Separating Past from Present**: Remind yourself that past situations do not have to define your current life. Therapy or counseling can help you break old emotional patterns.

Self-Worth vs. Validation from Others

One of the biggest traps is depending on external approval to feel valuable. After a breakup, you might try to find quick reassurance from friends or new dates. While praise can be nice, it is not a stable foundation. Real self-worth grows from your own acceptance of who you are.

- **Outside Compliments**: They can boost your mood but should not be your main source of confidence.
- **Building Internal Security**: This involves trusting your own judgement, recognizing your strengths, and knowing you are a complete person on your own.

Activities That Boost Self-Worth

1. **Learn a New Skill**
    - This can be anything from a language to a craft. Achieving small milestones in a new skill can remind you that you are capable.
2. **Physical Movement**
    - Yoga or simple body stretches can help you connect to your body, often increasing respect for what your body can do.
3. **Volunteering**
    - Helping others can give a sense of purpose. It shows that you have something to offer the world.
4. **Public Speaking**
    - Challenging yourself to speak in front of others, even in small groups, can build confidence in your voice and ideas.

Stopping Negative Thought Loops

- **Thought Journaling**: Each day, note recurring negative beliefs. Then rewrite them in a kinder way.
- **No Over-Identification**: If you think, "I fail at everything," ask yourself, "Is that really true, or is it just this situation?"
- **Focus on Present Facts**: Instead of letting your imagination run wild, look at what is actually happening. For instance, if you tried a new recipe and

it did not turn out well, that does not mean you are a bad cook forever. It just means the recipe needs adjusting or more practice.

Handling Social Media Triggers

After heartbreak, seeing others in happy relationships online can chip away at your self-worth even more. You might also see your ex posting about their life, which can be painful.

- **Unfollow or Mute**: If certain accounts trigger feelings of inferiority, there is no shame in muting them.
- **Reality Check**: Remember that social media often shows only highlights. People rarely post their struggles.
- **Time Limit**: Set a daily time limit for social media to protect your mental space.

Healing Through Giving Yourself Credit

If you are used to self-criticism, it feels unnatural to give yourself praise. But it is important to notice and acknowledge good choices or small wins. This is not about bragging; it is about balancing the negative thoughts you might have.

- **Mini-Celebrations**: If you completed a daunting task or overcame a bad day without sinking into self-blame, take a moment to note it. You could write a short sentence: "I handled that well."
- **Gratitude for Self**: Thank yourself for the effort you put in. This might be as simple as, "Thank you, self, for showing courage today."

Surprising Methods to Boost Self-Worth

1. **Mirror Accountability**
    - Stand in front of a mirror and state one thing you did right that day. Focus on your reflection as you say it out loud. This can feel odd at first, but it can help anchor positive words.
2. **Fasting from Negative Words**

- Challenge yourself not to use negative words about yourself for 24 hours. If you catch yourself saying, "I'm so dumb," stop, correct it with a gentler statement: "I made a mistake, but I can learn."
3. **Self-Worth Calendar**
    - Create a calendar where each day you write one positive thing about yourself. Over a month, you will have a growing list of qualities and actions that remind you that you have value.
4. **Daily Posture Check**
    - Slouching can worsen feelings of low worth. Straighten your back, pull your shoulders down, and lift your head. This physical shift can affect your mood.

Addressing Deep Guilt or Shame

Sometimes low self-worth is tied to guilt—maybe you wronged your partner, or you contributed to arguments in the relationship. While it is important to own mistakes, punishing yourself endlessly does not help.

- **Apologize if Needed**: If there is a real need for an apology, do it sincerely. Afterward, focus on how you can avoid repeating the mistake.
- **Practical Steps**: If you lied or acted poorly, figure out a plan for better behavior next time. This shows you are learning from your errors, not allowing them to define you.
- **Self-Forgiveness**: Remind yourself that everyone is capable of messing up. Growth is more important than dwelling on past errors forever.

Stepping Away from People Who Harm Your Self-Worth

In some cases, heartbreak comes with a circle of people who might gossip or take sides. If these people undermine your sense of self, consider limiting contact.

- **Identify Toxic Dynamics**: Do you leave conversations with certain friends or relatives feeling worse about yourself?
- **Set Boundaries**: This might mean shorter phone calls or responding less to negative messages. You do not have to explain yourself in detail. A simple "I need some space right now" can work.

- **Build a Healthier Network**: Look for friendships or groups that uplift you. This could be hobby clubs, support groups, or online communities focused on positivity.

Integrating New Habits Into Daily Life

You cannot rebuild self-worth in a single day. It requires consistent effort. Here are ways to weave self-worth exercises into your routine:

- **Morning Ritual**: Right after you wake up, say one kind thing to yourself. This can set a positive tone for the day.
- **Midday Reminder**: Place a sticky note with a positive affirmation on your computer or desk. When you glance at it, read it silently.
- **Evening Reflection**: Before bed, note one thing you did that shows you are trying to be kinder to yourself or more confident in your abilities.

What If Progress Feels Slow?

Rebuilding self-worth can be slow, especially if your heartbreak was severe or you have a long history of low confidence. It is normal to have ups and downs.

- **Be Patient**: Patience is crucial. Self-worth is like a muscle—regular practice makes it stronger.
- **Celebrate Small Shifts**: If a prohibited word is "celebrate," consider using "recognize" or "acknowledge." So, acknowledge small positive shifts. Notice if you handle a stressful event with less self-criticism than before.
- **Self-Compassion Over Perfection**: Nobody does this perfectly. Expect setbacks, but keep going. Each day, you can try again.

When to Seek Professional Support

Sometimes heartbreak triggers a deeper depression or long-term anxiety. You might feel stuck or unable to break free from harmful thoughts.

- **Therapy or Counseling**: A professional can teach tools specifically for low self-worth and heartbreak. They can also identify deeper issues that need attention.
- **Support Groups**: Whether in-person or online, these groups let you share experiences and hear how others cope.
- **Mental Health Hotlines**: If you feel overwhelmed or have thoughts of harming yourself, reach out for help immediately.

The Link Between Self-Worth and Future Relationships

A strong sense of self-worth affects all parts of your life, including future romantic connections. If you enter a new bond feeling worthless, you might put up with poor treatment or seek approval constantly. On the other hand, a healthy self-view helps you set boundaries and value respect.

- **Setting Standards**: Knowing your worth means you will not settle for less. You will be more aware of red flags or unhealthy patterns.
- **Healthy Communication**: A person who values themselves speaks honestly about needs and feelings.
- **Resilience**: Even if a future relationship ends, you will be better equipped to handle the disappointment because you have learned you are more than a relationship status.

Keeping Momentum

Strengthening self-worth is not a one-time project. It is ongoing maintenance of your mental and emotional health.

- **Review Progress Monthly**: Take a few minutes once a month to ask: "Do I feel better about myself now than I did a month ago?" If not, what small changes can you make?
- **Reward Growth**: Give yourself credit for any positive change, no matter how minor it may seem.
- **Stay Open to Growth**: Even when you feel more confident, remain open to learning. Life will present new challenges, and your self-worth skills will continue to evolve.

Conclusion of Chapter 6

Losing self-worth after heartbreak is a common experience, but it does not have to become your permanent truth. You can rebuild confidence by identifying your strengths, practicing positive self-talk, and limiting harmful influences. Day by day, small actions can restore your sense of value, reminding you that a breakup does not erase your worth.

In upcoming chapters, we will address more ways to care for yourself, manage outside pressures, and create a life that feels fulfilling on your own terms. You do not need a relationship to confirm your value—you already have qualities and abilities that make you an important person. By taking the steps outlined here, you will gradually see yourself with more kindness and respect, which sets the stage for healthier relationships in the future.

Chapter 7: Self-Care Basics for Emotional Pain

Heartbreak can make it hard to function from day to day. You may feel extreme sadness one moment, anger the next, and apathy soon after. When you are stuck in a tough emotional spot, it is easy to ignore your own well-being. But this is the time when looking after yourself is most important. Self-care does not have to be expensive or complicated. It involves giving your body and mind what they need to heal and restore balance.

This chapter focuses on practical methods of self-care that you can adapt to your own situation. We will talk about emotional, mental, and physical self-care, as well as ideas that go beyond the usual advice. Even small acts can help you feel calmer and more in control.

---

1. Defining Self-Care

Self-care is any action you take to maintain or improve your personal well-being. It is not about being selfish or ignoring other people's needs. Instead, it is about making sure you have the mental, physical, and emotional resources to handle life's challenges—especially heartbreak.

- **Mental Self-Care**: This involves managing stress, soothing anxious thoughts, and learning new mental skills to stay clear-headed.
- **Physical Self-Care**: Taking steps to keep the body in good shape, including proper rest, nutrition, and exercise.
- **Emotional Self-Care**: Handling your own feelings in ways that promote long-term healing, such as journaling or spending time with people who uplift you.

---

2. Why Self-Care Feels Hard After Heartbreak

When sadness weighs heavily, simple tasks can feel huge. You might feel it is too exhausting to cook a meal or go for a walk. Other times, you might think you do not "deserve" to feel better because the relationship ended. These thoughts can push you deeper into despair.

- **Low Motivation**: Heartbreak can steal your energy, leaving you feeling stuck.
- **Guilt**: You might blame yourself for the breakup and feel you do not have the right to be happy.
- **Misunderstanding of Self-Care**: Some people think self-care is selfish or a luxury, but it is actually a healthy practice for survival and wellness.

---

3. Starting with Simple Physical Self-Care

Taking care of your body can have a positive effect on your emotions. When your body feels stronger, your mind is more likely to cope with distress.

3.1. Gentle Nutrition

- **Snack on Whole Foods**: Include fruits, vegetables, nuts, and whole grains. These keep blood sugar steady, which can help prevent mood swings.
- **Hydration**: Drink enough water throughout the day. Dehydration can lead to headaches and fatigue, increasing negative moods.
- **Mindful Eating**: Pay attention to each bite. This reduces the chance of overeating or neglecting meals altogether.

3.2. Rest and Sleep

- **Steady Bedtime**: Going to bed around the same time each night helps stabilize your internal clock.
- **Screen-Free Hour**: Avoid screens (phone, TV, computer) before bed. The light from devices can interfere with sleep hormones.
- **Short Relaxation Ritual**: Try reading a calm book, doing light stretches, or writing down worries in a notebook before turning out the lights.

3.3. Light Exercise

- **Walking**: A 20-minute walk outside can clear your head and expose you to fresh air.
- **Simple Home Routines**: Even a few jumping jacks or a short yoga-like routine (gentle stretching) can release endorphins.

- **Dance to Music**: Put on a tune you enjoy, and move in any way that feels natural. This can ease tension from your muscles.

---

4. Emotional Self-Care Techniques

When heartbreak strikes, your emotions can feel like a roller coaster. Emotional self-care means giving yourself a healthy outlet for those intense feelings and offering your heart some extra gentleness.

4.1. Short Emotional Check-Ins

- **Set Timers**: Twice a day, pause whatever you are doing and ask, "How do I feel right now?"
- **Name the Emotion**: If you are sad, label it as sadness. If you are angry, label it as anger. This can reduce the power of the emotion.
- **Deep Breathing**: After naming the feeling, take three slow, deep breaths. Focus on the sensation of air moving in and out of your lungs.

4.2. Constructive Releases

- **Tearful Release**: Crying in a safe space can help. Many people feel relief after letting tears flow for a while.
- **Art Expression**: Painting, scribbling, or clay modeling can channel your sadness or anger into colors and shapes.
- **Singing or Humming**: As discussed in a previous chapter, singing can let you unload tension in your chest and throat.

4.3. Positive Distractions

- **Healthy Hobbies**: Engaging in crafts, reading a book, or learning a new skill can distract you from negative thoughts.
- **Simple Puzzles or Brain Teasers**: Crossword puzzles, sudoku, or word games can help shift your mind into problem-solving mode, reducing emotional overwhelm.

---

5. Mental Self-Care Tips

The mind often replays painful memories or questions about the breakup. Mental self-care involves guiding your thoughts in a more supportive direction.

5.1. Regulating Your Inner Voice

- **Challenge Harmful Thoughts**: If a thought says, "I am unlovable," ask, "Is that really true, or is it my sadness talking?"
- **Affirmations in Moderation**: Short phrases like "I can heal," "I have value," or "I will get through this" can replace negative beliefs if you repeat them regularly.
- **Set Mental Boundaries**: If you catch yourself stuck in a negative cycle, try a short activity—like drinking a glass of water or folding laundry—to break the loop.

5.2. Information Diet

- **Limit Sad Media**: Watching too many sad movies or listening to heartbreak songs all day might deepen your gloom. Choose media that uplifts you.
- **Avoid "Horror Stories"**: When heartbreak is fresh, hearing about other people's worst relationship woes can heighten your anxiety.
- **Focus on Constructive Material**: Books or podcasts about self-improvement, psychology, or hope can bring new perspectives.

---

6. Building a Self-Care Environment

Where you live or spend most of your time can shape how you feel. A cluttered, messy, or stressful environment might worsen heartbreak symptoms. A soothing environment can make you feel safer.

6.1. Simple Space Cleanup

- **Clear Surfaces**: Keep a table or desk free of clutter. This helps the mind feel less overwhelmed.
- **Wash the Dishes**: Even small tasks like washing dishes or taking out the trash can reduce mental clutter and build a sense of accomplishment.
- **Put Away Memory Triggers**: If certain items remind you too strongly of your ex-partner, store them out of sight while you heal.

6.2. Comfort Corners

- **Cozy Chair or Cushion**: Pick a spot in your home for relaxation, reading, or journaling. Keep it clean and comfortable.

- **Soft Lighting**: Bright overhead lights can feel harsh. Lamps or fairy lights can create a calmer mood.
- **Music or Nature Sounds**: Play calming music or natural sounds (rain, ocean waves) in the background when you are resting.

---

7. Time Management for Self-Care

When you feel sad, it is easy to get lost in aimless scrolling on social media or lying in bed for hours. While rest is important, structuring your day can help you avoid being swallowed by negative thoughts.

7.1. Simple Routines

- **Morning Routine**: Wake up at a set time, wash your face, and drink a glass of water. This signals your body that a new day has begun.
- **Midday Check-In**: Use lunch as a reminder to ask yourself how you are feeling. Do you need to step outside for a moment?
- **Evening Wind-Down**: Reserve the last half-hour before bedtime for calm activities like gentle stretching, reading, or writing your thoughts in a journal.

7.2. Scheduling Breaks

- **Micro-Breaks**: Every hour, take a 1-minute break to close your eyes or stand up and stretch.
- **Mini Self-Care Sessions**: Set aside 10-15 minutes a couple of times a day for quick self-care: make a cup of herbal tea, listen to a soothing song, or do a short breathing exercise.

---

8. Social Aspects of Self-Care

While self-care focuses on you, it does not mean shutting out everyone else. The people in your life can be resources—or they can add stress. Being aware of who you spend time with and how they affect you is part of self-care.

8.1. Selective Socializing

- **Plan Time with Supportive Friends**: Invite someone you trust to watch a light-hearted show or share a meal.
- **Limit Negative Interactions**: If you have friends who constantly bring drama or cause you to question yourself, consider reducing the time you spend with them, at least during the most fragile phase of your heartbreak.
- **Consider Group Activities**: Sometimes, participating in a group activity (like a local club or hobby group) can help you feel connected without having to talk about your personal issues too much.

8.2. Setting Boundaries

- **Saying "No"**: If someone invites you to an event you do not feel ready for, it is okay to politely decline.
- **Careful with Advice-Givers**: Everyone may have opinions on how you should handle your breakup. You can thank them for their concern but still make your own decisions.
- **Guard Your Quiet Time**: If you need alone time to decompress, let people know in advance.

---

9. Uncommon Self-Care Ideas (Golden Insights)

Here are some less-talked-about approaches to self-care that might offer a fresh perspective:

1. **Laughter Exercises**
   - Even forced laughter can trigger a chemical reaction in the brain that lifts mood. Look for short comedy clips, or just try laughing out loud for 30 seconds in private. It can feel silly, but sometimes it quickly eases stress.
2. **Grief Stones**
   - Find a small stone that fits in your hand. Hold it when you feel sad, let your negative thoughts flow into it, then place it back in a special box or on a shelf. This physical action can represent storing away some of your sorrow for a later time, giving you a small mental break.
3. **Random Acts of Kindness**

        - Helping strangers or acquaintances—like paying for someone's coffee or leaving a friendly note—can give you a sense of connection and purpose. This can boost your self-regard during painful times.
    4. **Mindful Coloring**
        - Adult coloring books exist for a reason. The repetitive motion of coloring detailed patterns can calm a racing mind. Even a few minutes can reduce overthinking.
    5. **Bath Time Ritual**
        - A warm bath with Epsom salts can help muscles relax. Light a candle, sip a warm drink, and allow yourself a short mental vacation. This can be a comforting form of self-care you might overlook.

---

10. Handling Setbacks and Guilt

You might try a self-care plan, only to miss a day or slip back into old habits. Remember that setbacks are normal. Healing from heartbreak is not a simple, straight line.

- **Be Kind to Yourself**: If you forget your routine or skip a walk, it does not mean you have failed. It means you are human.
- **Review and Adjust**: Maybe a certain activity felt too demanding. Try a smaller step or a different approach.
- **Do Not Compare**: Everyone heals at their own pace. Comparing your progress with someone else's can add unnecessary pressure.

---

11. Financial Self-Care

Money stress can make heartbreak even worse. While this will be covered more deeply in a later chapter (Chapter 17 about financial independence), a few basics can help right now:

- **Create a Simple Budget**: List your monthly income and regular expenses. Seeing the numbers on paper can reduce anxiety.

- **Cut Unnecessary Spending**: Temporary heartbreak shopping may feel good in the moment but can cause guilt later. Set a small allowance for "fun purchases" and stick to it.
- **Plan for the Future**: If you shared bills or an apartment with your ex, you may need to adjust your budget to handle living on your own. Seek financial advice if needed.

12. Digital Self-Care Boundaries

The internet can be a source of both comfort and stress.

- **Mute the Ex**: If seeing your ex's social media posts hurts you, consider unfollowing or blocking them, at least temporarily.
- **Screen-Free Blocks of Time**: Dedicate certain hours of the day to be offline. This can lower the emotional overload from constant notifications.
- **Mindful Browsing**: Before you click on a story or watch a video, ask yourself if it will help or harm your current state of mind.

13. Long-Term Mindset for Self-Care

Self-care during heartbreak is not just about feeling better momentarily. It builds habits that can support you for the rest of your life. When you care for your body, mind, and emotions, you set the stage for healthier relationships and a more balanced approach to life's ups and downs.

- **Consistency Over Perfection**: It is better to do a little self-care every day than to wait until you are completely drained.
- **Evolving Needs**: As you heal, the ways you care for yourself might change. You may move from quiet reflection to more active pursuits.
- **Self-Awareness**: Over time, you will learn the signs of emotional strain and can respond earlier with effective self-care.

14. Putting It All Together

Self-care is a combination of small daily steps. You do not have to transform your life overnight. Start with one or two strategies that feel easy and gradually add more. You might keep a checklist or planner where you note each day's self-care actions (e.g., "Went for a walk," "Drank enough water," "Talked to a friend").

Remember, heartbreak can drain you, making everything feel heavier. But self-care lights the path to emotional stability. By choosing to look after your body, mind, and heart, you confirm that your well-being matters, even if a relationship has ended.

Chapter 7 Conclusion

Self-care provides the fuel you need to get through the pain of heartbreak. It covers simple habits like resting well, eating balanced meals, engaging in moderate exercise, and finding outlets for emotional stress. Beyond that, you can shape your environment, manage your time, and explore less common methods (like laughter exercises or holding "grief stones") to find relief. There is no one-size-fits-all plan for self-care, so experiment with different methods until you discover what works.

In the next chapter, we will look at how to ask for help and support from the people around you. Although self-care is a personal responsibility, nobody is meant to endure heartbreak completely alone. There are times when outside help can make all the difference.

Chapter 8: How to Ask for Help and Support

Heartbreak often feels isolating. You might think, "Nobody understands exactly what I am going through." Or you may worry that reaching out will make you a burden. Yet, seeking help is a crucial part of healing. Humans are social creatures, and many of our emotional struggles respond well to understanding and empathy from others.

This chapter explores why asking for help is challenging for some, how to find the right people to lean on, and strategies for forming a supportive network. We will also cover when professional help might be needed. Remember, asking for support does not mean you are weak; it shows you are wise enough to recognize you do not have to face heartbreak alone.

---

1. Understanding the Fear of Reaching Out

1. **Fear of Judgment**
    - You might think others will blame you for the breakup or see you as a failure. This worry can stop you from sharing your feelings.
2. **Pride or Independence**
    - Some individuals were taught to handle problems on their own. They feel that asking for help shows weakness or immaturity.
3. **Past Disappointments**
    - If friends or family have let you down before, you may hesitate to trust them again or believe that support is even possible.
4. **Guilt Over Burdening Others**
    - You might feel that everyone else is busy with their own lives. This guilt can make you reluctant to speak up about your pain.

---

2. Reasons You Should Ask for Help

1. **Shared Experience**
    - Many people have gone through breakups. They can offer insights or at least a listening ear.
2. **Emotional Relief**

- Talking about your heartbreak can lighten your emotional load. Keeping everything inside often makes it feel heavier.
3. **New Perspectives**
    - A friend or counselor can point out options you had not considered or remind you of your strengths.
4. **Practical Support**
    - Beyond emotional help, others might assist with tasks like moving, cooking meals, or watching your kids if you are a parent.

---

3. Identifying Who Can Support You

Not everyone in your life is well-suited to give the help you need. It is important to choose people who are genuinely caring and trustworthy.

3.1. Types of Supporters

- **Close Friends**: People you have known for a while and who understand you deeply.
- **Family Members**: Relatives who are patient, kind, and willing to listen.
- **Colleagues or Classmates**: Sometimes, a coworker or fellow student can be surprisingly supportive, especially if they are empathetic or have faced a breakup themselves.
- **Support Groups**: Groups of people who share similar experiences, usually guided by a leader or just meeting informally.
- **Counselors or Therapists**: Professionals with training to help people heal from emotional distress.

3.2. Evaluating Reliability

- **Do They Keep Confidences?**: You want someone who will not spread your private details.
- **Are They Good Listeners?**: Some folks prefer to talk about themselves and do not give you space to speak.
- **Do They Show Empathy?**: Empathy means they try to understand how you feel without rushing to judge or fix you.

4. How to Ask for Help

Many people feel awkward when trying to ask for emotional support. They might downplay their pain or say, "I'm sorry to bother you, but…" Here are some clearer ways to approach people:

1. **Be Direct**
   - "I am going through a hard time right now, and I would really appreciate someone to talk to."
2. **Share a Bit of Context**
   - You do not have to lay out every detail. A short summary like "My relationship ended, and I'm struggling with sadness" can help the other person understand what you need.
3. **Specify the Kind of Help**
   - Are you just looking for a listening ear? Do you need practical help, like running errands? Let them know.
4. **Offer Flexibility**
   - Ask if there is a good time for them to talk or meet. This shows respect for their schedule.

---

5. Setting Boundaries When Receiving Help

Asking for help does not mean you have to agree to every suggestion or question. You remain in control of your own story.

- **You Choose What to Share**: You do not have to reveal every single detail if it makes you uncomfortable.
- **Limit Advice Overload**: If you feel bombarded by too many suggestions, let the person know: "I appreciate your ideas, but I really just need to vent right now."
- **Keep Emotional Safety**: If someone starts judging or blaming you, it is okay to gently end the conversation or shift the topic.

---

6. Overcoming Common Hurdles

6.1. Feeling Undeserving of Help

You might think, "Others have bigger problems than mine." This comparison can make you feel like you do not deserve support. Remember that everyone's pain is valid. Heartbreak can be just as intense as any other crisis.

6.2. Not Wanting to Appear Vulnerable

Being open about your feelings can be scary. But true connection often happens when we allow ourselves to be real. Bottling up everything might create a hard shell, but it also keeps warmth and understanding at a distance.

6.3. Dealing with Letdowns

Sometimes, people you trust might not respond how you hope. They could be too busy, or they might not understand the depth of your pain. Do not let one letdown stop you from seeking help elsewhere.

---

7. Professional Help: When and Why

Sometimes, family and friends are not enough. You might need a trained professional who can guide you more carefully through heartbreak.

7.1. Signs You Might Need Professional Support

- **Prolonged Sadness**: Feeling sad most of the time for weeks or months without improvement.
- **Harmful Thoughts**: If you think about hurting yourself or giving up on life.
- **Physical or Anxiety Issues**: Heart palpitations, panic attacks, or severe insomnia triggered by emotional distress.
- **Repeated Harmful Relationship Patterns**: You notice you keep choosing partners who hurt you or that you sabotage every relationship.

7.2. Types of Professionals

- **Counselors/Therapists**: Trained to help with emotional healing, relationship issues, and coping strategies.

- **Psychologists**: Often have advanced training in diagnosing mental health challenges and can offer talk therapy.
- **Psychiatrists**: Medical doctors who can diagnose conditions and prescribe medication if needed, though not every heartbreak needs medication.
- **Support Group Leaders**: Sometimes found in group therapy settings or community programs.

---

8. Using Technology to Find Support

We live in a digital era where help can be found online. However, it is important to be careful about which online sources you use.

8.1. Online Support Groups or Forums

- **Anonymous Sharing**: You can often post your story without revealing your real name.
- **Varied Perspectives**: People from around the world might comment, giving you a broad range of advice.
- **Cautions**: Some places might have negative or toxic discussions. If you find the group is too harsh or you feel worse after reading posts, look for a different one.

8.2. Telehealth Counseling

- **Video or Phone Sessions**: You can speak with a counselor from home. This can be helpful if you have mobility issues or live in an area with limited in-person services.
- **Scheduling Ease**: Appointments can be more flexible.
- **Insurance Coverage**: Check if your insurance or local programs cover telehealth therapy.

---

9. The Role of Faith or Spiritual Communities

For those who have a religious or spiritual background, places of worship or faith-based groups can offer a network of compassionate people. Some religious leaders are open to offering guidance or just listening. It is important to seek a community or leader who respects your feelings and offers comfort instead of blame.

10. How to Give People Helpful Feedback

When you ask for help, the people you confide in may try their best, but they might not always say or do the right thing. It is okay to let them know what type of support works best for you.

- **Compliment the Good**: If your friend or family member says something helpful, let them know: "That really helped me feel understood."
- **Guide Them Gently**: If they start lecturing you, consider saying, "I just need someone to hear me right now, not fix the problem."
- **Be Honest**: Sometimes friends and family do not realize their well-intentioned advice can feel hurtful or rushed. Explaining your feelings can help them adjust.

11. Balancing Between Sharing and Relying Too Much

It is healthy to share your burdens, but be mindful of not transferring all your emotional weight onto one person. Friendships can get strained if one friend constantly listens without any break. Try to distribute your needs among different sources of support:

- **Varied Sources**: Talk to different friends, attend a support group, and maybe see a counselor. Spread the emotional load.
- **Offer Something Back**: Ask about your friend's life, too. Even a small act of caring for them shows that you appreciate their time and are not only focused on your own issues.

12. Uncommon Methods of Seeking Help (Golden Insights)

1. **Shared Interest Meetups**
    - Join groups or classes for an activity you like—cooking, hiking, photography. Even if you do not talk about heartbreak openly,

connecting over shared interests can help you make new friends and feel less alone.
   2. **"Listening Partner" Agreement**
      - Arrange with a trusted friend that you will take turns listening to each other's problems for a set period (like 10 minutes each). This structure avoids one-sided vents and ensures both parties get time to talk.
   3. **Anonymous Phone Lines**
      - Some countries have hotlines where you can call and speak to a listener or counselor for free. This can be a quick way to unburden yourself in times of extreme sadness or if you have no one else to talk to.
   4. **Spiritual Retreats or Workshops**
      - If you are open to it, certain retreats or workshops focus on personal reflection. They often have trained leaders who guide participants through healing exercises, meditation, or quiet time.

---

13. Handling Responses You Dislike

Not everyone will respond well when you ask for support. They might give misguided advice, judge you, or dismiss your feelings. This does not invalidate your need for help.

- **Reject the Message, Not Yourself**: If someone says, "You should just get over it," that is their ignorance talking. It does not mean your pain is less real.
- **Set Firm Boundaries**: If they repeatedly belittle you or pry too much into your personal details, you have the right to end the conversation.
- **Redirect to Someone Else**: Seek out a friend, counselor, or group that shows genuine empathy.

---

14. Practical Steps for Group Support

Support groups can be especially helpful if they are well-run. Here's how to get the most out of them:

- **Find the Right Fit**: Look for a group that focuses on heartbreak recovery or emotional wellness. Read reviews or ask about the group's rules to ensure it is a respectful place.
- **Arrive with an Open Mind**: You might hear others' stories that differ from yours. Value their experiences but remember everyone's path is unique.
- **Listen Actively**: You can gain insight from hearing how others cope, even if their situation is not exactly like yours.
- **Contribute Slowly**: If you are shy, you can start by just listening. Over time, you may feel comfortable sharing.

15. When Family Isn't Supportive

In some cultures or families, heartbreak might be treated as a private matter, or there may be shame around discussing personal problems. If your family is unsupportive or scolds you for sharing, consider alternative support channels.

- **Build Your "Chosen Family"**: Surround yourself with friends or mentors who act like family in how they care for you.
- **Seek Professional Outlets**: Counselors, group therapy, or online communities can offer what your family cannot.
- **Minimal Disclosure**: You can limit what you tell your family if their reactions tend to worsen your emotional state.

16. Encouraging Yourself to Keep Asking

Persistence matters. You might ask a friend for help on a bad day and feel better, but heartbreak often returns in waves. It is okay to seek support again on another rough day. Make sure you:

- **Avoid Apologizing Excessively**: You can say "Thank you for listening" rather than "I'm sorry I'm bothering you again."
- **Spread It Out**: If you worry about burdening one person too much, alternate between different supportive friends or resources.
- **Acknowledge Their Effort**: A simple "I appreciate your time" or "Your help means a lot to me" can strengthen these bonds.

17. Strength in Shared Healing

Sometimes the best form of help is just knowing you are not alone. Sharing heartbreak stories with friends or in safe online spaces can be therapeutic. Hearing someone else say, "I felt the same way last year, and now I'm doing better," can spark hope that your pain is temporary.

- **No Pressure to Heal Immediately**: Everyone's timeline is different. You can keep seeking support until you reach a state of stability.
- **Pay It Forward**: In the future, you might be the person someone else turns to when they face heartbreak. Your experience can guide them.

---

18. Maintaining a Support Network Over Time

Once the intense pain of heartbreak subsides, do not forget the people who stood by you. Maintaining these bonds can provide ongoing emotional security. Offer support in return if they ever need it.

- **Check In Regularly**: Send a quick message or plan occasional meetups.
- **Share Good News**: Let them know when you have made progress or feel better, so they can see that their help mattered.
- **Stay Connected**: Even if you are no longer in crisis, keep your support system close. You never know when life's challenges might appear again.

---

19. Creating a Plan for Support

To make asking for help more straightforward, you can prepare a simple plan or "support roadmap":

1. **List Possible Helpers**: Friends, family, colleagues, professionals.
2. **Note Their Strengths**: Which one is a good listener? Who might help with practical tasks?
3. **Set Contact Preferences**: Some people are best reached by text, others prefer a call or face-to-face meetings.
4. **Create a Backup**: If the first person you call is unavailable, have a second or third choice lined up. This reduces panic or the urge to isolate yourself.

20. Conclusion of Chapter 8

Asking for help after heartbreak is a powerful choice. It shows that you understand healing is not a solo effort. You deserve comfort, guidance, and empathy as you work through the pain. Whether you turn to trusted friends, family members, professionals, or online groups, the key is to reach out in ways that feel right for you.

Remember, heartbreak can sometimes cloud your ability to see that people do care. By letting them into your world, you open doors to fresh ideas, emotional relief, and practical solutions. In the upcoming chapters, we will look at rebuilding trust in yourself, learning from your past, and many more steps you can take to shape a healthier future. Your willingness to ask for support sets the stage for ongoing healing and growth—proving that even in the worst times, you do not have to stand alone.

Chapter 9: Rebuilding Trust in Yourself

When you experience heartbreak, you can lose not only trust in the other person but also trust in your own ability to make good decisions. You might look back at the red flags you missed or the warnings you brushed aside and think, "How could I have been so blind?" This doubt can eat away at your confidence, making you question your judgment in future situations.

Rebuilding trust in yourself is essential if you want to move forward in a healthy way. This chapter focuses on practical steps to regain the confidence that you can handle life's ups and downs without fear that you will repeat past mistakes. You will learn strategies for examining what went wrong, how to accept your humanity, and how to take measured risks that build your sense of security.

---

1. Understanding Self-Trust

Self-trust is the belief that you can rely on your instincts, reasoning, and moral compass. It does not mean you will never err again. It means you trust yourself to deal with challenges, learn from mistakes, and adapt if your chosen path does not work out perfectly.

When heartbreak occurs, it is common to lose some level of faith in yourself. You might think, "I should have seen it coming," or, "I always choose the wrong people." These thoughts produce self-doubt that can linger, especially if you have had multiple painful breakups.

- **Emotional Security**: Self-trust provides internal safety. Even when things are uncertain, you know you can fall back on your internal judgment.
- **Decision-Making Power**: When you trust yourself, you do not get stuck in a loop of asking others for approval. You can weigh options and feel good about your choices, even if they are not guaranteed to succeed.
- **Freedom from Self-Punishment**: People who lack self-trust often punish themselves with negative self-talk. Rebuilding trust loosens that pattern, letting you approach life with more kindness toward yourself.

---

2. Why Self-Trust Often Breaks After Heartbreak

1. **Ignoring Red Flags**
   - Maybe you saw signs of dishonesty or disrespect but chose to ignore them, believing the situation would improve. Afterward, you might label yourself foolish and wonder why you did not act sooner.
   - This can lead to self-criticism: "If I could not see something that obvious, I must be bad at reading people."
2. **Guilt Over Personal Mistakes**
   - If you contributed to relationship problems—maybe through harmful words, jealousy, or emotional distance—you might assume you will repeat these behaviors in the future.
   - This guilt can create shame that blocks your confidence in your own growth and willingness to do better next time.
3. **External Criticism**
   - Sometimes friends or family blame you for the breakup. Even if they are not entirely correct, their words can sink into your mind: "You drove them away," or "You did not make enough effort."
   - Over time, you may start to believe these negative opinions, causing further damage to your self-trust.
4. **Confusion Between Trusting Others vs. Trusting Yourself**
   - It is easy to mix up the idea of trusting other people with trusting your own judgment. If your ex-partner lied or betrayed you, you might unconsciously conclude that it was your error for trusting them. You might start believing you are incapable of discerning who is trustworthy and who is not.

---

3. The Cost of Living Without Self-Trust

When self-trust is damaged, everyday life can become a minefield of indecision and insecurity:

- **Fear of Making Choices**: You might hesitate over small decisions—like what to wear, where to go, or which job to apply for—because you are worried about "messing up" again.

- **Seeking Constant Approval**: Without internal reassurance, you might rely on friends, family, or even random online opinions to feel comfortable in your decisions.
- **Self-Sabotage**: If you believe you always fail, you might shy away from new relationships or sabotage them the moment issues appear.
- **Missed Opportunities**: Lack of self-trust can stop you from taking steps that might lead to personal growth, such as moving to a new city, starting a business, or entering a new social circle.

---

4. First Steps to Rebuild Trust in Yourself

4.1. Honest Self-Reflection

Take time to examine the role you played in the relationship and the signs you might have overlooked. This is not about punishing yourself—it is about understanding your patterns.

- **Write It Down**: In a notebook, list what you did well (e.g., loyalty, open communication) and where you might have dropped the ball (e.g., ignoring your own boundaries, refusing to speak up when something bothered you).
- **Stay Balanced**: Acknowledge that no relationship ends solely because of one person. Even if your ex was primarily at fault, you can learn something about how you respond to conflict or deception.

4.2. Accepting Your Humanity

You are not a machine. Every human being misses warning signs sometimes or becomes too hopeful. Recognizing that "I made a mistake, but that does not define my entire self" is crucial.

- **Self-Compassion Phrases**: Practice saying, "I am learning," "I am growing," or "I made a mistake, but I can improve."
- **Dropping the All-or-Nothing Mindset**: Instead of "I always mess up," try, "I made errors in that relationship, but I also did many things right."

4.3. Gathering Evidence of Your Past Successes

Self-trust is not only about heartbreak situations. Look at other areas of life where you have shown good judgment or problem-solving skills:

- **Professional Achievements**: Maybe you managed a project at work or navigated a tough financial situation.
- **Personal Trials**: Look at times you overcame health issues or personal struggles. You may have been resourceful in finding solutions or adapting.
- **Daily Victories**: Even small decisions—like helping a friend solve a problem or choosing a new recipe that turned out well—count as evidence that you can handle life's uncertainties.

---

5. Practical Exercises to Strengthen Self-Trust

5.1. Small Decision Challenges

Often, heartbreak shakes your faith in making big relationship decisions. But you can rebuild trust in smaller ways first:

1. **Pick a Simple Goal**: Choose a minor area in your life—like deciding on a new hobby or rearranging your living room furniture—and commit to a plan.
2. **Follow Through**: Even if you are uncertain, see it to the end. Notice how you handled bumps along the way.
3. **Reflect on Results**: If it worked out, celebrate mentally by saying, "I can do this." If it did not work out, identify what you learned and still praise yourself for taking action.

5.2. Listening to Intuition

Sometimes heartbreak makes you doubt your instincts. Try short exercises to reconnect with your gut feeling:

- **Moment of Stillness**: Sit quietly for a few minutes. Ask yourself a simple question like, "What do I feel like eating today?" or, "Do I need rest or activity right now?" Listen to your internal answer before logic and doubts rush in.
- **Track Intuitive Hits**: Keep a small journal of each time you followed your intuition and what happened. Over weeks, you may see a pattern that reminds you your instincts can be valuable.

5.3. "What If I Am Right?" Method

When a fearful thought shows up—like, "What if I pick the wrong person again?"—flip it around by asking, "What if I pick a healthier partner this time because I have learned from my past?"

- **Direct Your Mind**: This technique helps you see that the future is not fixed. You have grown, so your outcomes can be different.
- **Focus on the Good Outcome**: Even if it does not erase worry, it balances out the negative assumptions with a positive possibility.

---

6. Handling the Inner Critic

Heartbreak can unleash a loud inner critic that mocks your attempts to trust yourself. This critic might say, "You are naïve," or, "You will fail again." While you cannot silence it completely, you can learn to manage it:

- **Recognize Its Voice**: Notice when these harsh thoughts appear. Label them: "That is my inner critic."
- **Respond with Reason**: Counter the critic's statements. If it says, "You always choose the worst partners," remind yourself, "That was one relationship (or two). I have the power to make better choices now."
- **Limit Its Frequency**: Sometimes writing the critic's statements on a piece of paper and then throwing it away can symbolize rejecting destructive self-talk.

---

7. Learning Assertiveness

Trusting yourself also means speaking up for your needs and values. If you have had a pattern of ignoring your gut feelings in relationships, assertiveness can be a game-changer.

7.1. Define Your Boundaries

- **Identify Areas of Discomfort**: Did you let your ex treat you poorly? Did you agree to things you were not comfortable with? Make a list of non-negotiable boundaries (e.g., no yelling, no insults, no ignoring).

- **Decide What Consequences Follow**: If someone crosses these boundaries, how will you respond? You might give a warning or end the interaction.

7.2. Practice Saying "No"

- **Start Small**: Say "no" to minor requests you do not have time or energy for. This builds your ability to assert your needs without guilt.
- **Steer Clear of Over-Explaining**: A simple, "I can't do that right now," or, "That doesn't work for me," is enough. Trust that you have the right to set limits.

---

8. Gradual Exposure to Relationship-Related Situations

If heartbreak shook your self-trust in the context of romance, it might be hard to imagine dating again or even flirting with someone new. Gradual exposure allows you to re-engage with social situations at a pace that feels manageable.

8.1. Casual Social Interactions

- **Group Outings**: Participate in group events where the pressure is low. Observe how you feel around potential new people.
- **Short Conversations**: Practice talking to someone you find interesting for a few minutes, then step away if you feel overwhelmed. Over time, you can extend these interactions.

8.2. Healthy Boundaries in Early Dating

- **Define Red Flags**: Make a list of behaviors or traits that are deal-breakers for you based on your past experiences (e.g., consistent lying, disrespect, ignoring your feelings).
- **Stick to It**: If you notice one of these red flags, trust yourself enough to walk away early before investing too heavily in the connection.

---

9. Seeking Validation in Healthy Ways

There is a difference between healthy validation and complete dependence on external approval. Healthy validation is when you listen to feedback and use it to refine your perspective, without letting it override your intuition.

- **Ask for Input, Not Permission**: You might say to a friend, "What do you think of this situation?" rather than, "Tell me what to do."
- **Value Balanced Opinions**: Seek out people who respect your autonomy and do not push their agenda on you.
- **Recognize Toxic Validation**: If someone consistently invalidates your feelings or demands you follow their guidance, that is not healthy input.

---

10. Overcoming the Fear of Repeating Mistakes

It is normal to worry that you will fall into the same pattern. This worry itself can be a barrier to trusting your future decisions.

10.1. Reflect, Do Not Ruminate

Reflecting means calmly looking at what happened and noting lessons. Ruminating means going in circles with no new insights.

- **Set Time Limits**: Give yourself 15 minutes to think about the breakup or your fears, then move on to another activity.
- **Focus on Growth**: Each time you review the past, identify at least one thing you can do differently in the future.

10.2. Reward Self-Awareness

When you catch yourself approaching a familiar problem with a new strategy, acknowledge it:

- **Example**: You notice someone you recently met has a pattern of only texting you at odd hours, ignoring your messages for days. Before, you might have justified it. Now, you set a boundary or voice your concern. Recognize that as progress.

---

11. Recognizing Small Wins

Building self-trust does not happen overnight. You gain it gradually through experiences that confirm your reliability toward yourself.

1. **Mini Victories**: When you make a decision—such as choosing a weekend activity or planning a short trip—and it works out well, mentally say, "I made a good call."
2. **Resilience in Face of Mistakes**: Even if a decision does not lead to a perfect outcome, note how you handled it. If you stayed calm and tried to fix the problem, that is a sign of growth.
3. **Building a Track Record**: Over time, these small wins accumulate. You begin to have a record of times you acted based on your judgment, and life did not fall apart.

---

12. Visualization Exercises

Sometimes you need to see yourself as a trustworthy person before you can fully live it out. Visualization can help:

- **Calm Space**: Sit or lie down in a quiet area, close your eyes, and breathe slowly.
- **Picture Yourself**: Imagine yourself in a situation that used to scare you—maybe confronting someone who disrespects you or calmly walking away from a toxic person.
- **Feel the Outcome**: In your mind, see yourself staying confident, speaking clearly, and then feeling proud afterward. This mental rehearsal can build readiness for real-life encounters.

---

13. Addressing Deeper Emotional Wounds

In some cases, you may have deeper issues tied to childhood or past traumas that make self-trust especially difficult. If heartbreak triggers memories of abandonment or other serious wounds, professional help might be the best way forward.

- **Therapy or Counseling**: A trained counselor can help you identify subconscious beliefs that keep you from trusting yourself.
- **Support Groups**: Groups for survivors of emotional abuse or betrayal can offer community support and coping strategies.
- **Self-Help Books or Resources**: Books on trauma recovery or self-confidence might give you structured exercises to heal deeper layers of doubt.

14. Physical Actions That Promote Self-Trust

While self-trust is mental and emotional, sometimes physical exercises can support it:

- **Posture Checks**: Standing up straight, shoulders relaxed, and head held level can shift how you feel about yourself. Slouching often goes hand-in-hand with low self-esteem.
- **Physical Challenges**: Setting a goal like a 5K walk or a new workout routine—and following through—can teach you that you have discipline and resilience.
- **Adrenaline Activities**: If it is safe and you feel curious, trying something like indoor rock climbing or a ropes course can show you that you are braver than you assume.

---

15. Creating a "Self-Trust Menu"

One practical idea is to create a "menu" of actions you can take whenever you feel self-doubt creeping in. This menu could be a short list on your phone or in a small notebook:

- **Affirmations**: "I am capable," "I am allowed to grow."
- **Short Grounding Practices**: 5 deep breaths, a 2-minute meditation, or stepping outside to look at the sky.
- **Reach Out to a Trusted Friend**: A quick text or call to someone who respects your autonomy.
- **Reflective Questions**: "Have I learned from my mistakes?" "What is the worst that could happen if I trust myself on this?"

Having this menu at hand can help you respond quickly when self-doubt appears, rather than sinking into anxious overthinking.

---

16. Celebrating (Acknowledging) Your Growth Without Guilt

You might feel uncomfortable accepting your own progress because you fear slipping back. But it is healthy to acknowledge growth as you go:

- **Mini Rewards**: If you handle a tough conversation well, treat yourself to something small you enjoy, like a warm bath or a favorite dessert. (Again, we avoid the restricted verb, simply calling it a "treat" or "reward.")
- **Share with Others**: Telling a trusted friend, "I faced my fear today!" can reinforce that sense of achievement.
- **Avoid Perfectionism**: You do not need to be perfect to note progress. Real life is messy, and partial improvements still count.

---

17. When Others Challenge Your Newfound Self-Trust

Sometimes, friends or family who are used to you doubting yourself might be unsettled when you start to stand firm. They might say, "You have changed," or accuse you of being arrogant. This can test your resolve.

- **Stand Your Ground**: Politely but firmly say, "I am trying a new way of taking care of myself. I appreciate your concern, but this is important to me."
- **Explain If Safe**: You might briefly share that you are learning to trust your own decisions after a difficult experience, but you do not owe anyone a detailed explanation if you do not wish to give one.
- **Beware Manipulation**: In some cases, if a person feels threatened by your growing confidence, they may try to undermine you. Notice that behavior and maintain your boundaries.

---

18. Recognizing Long-Term Benefits of Self-Trust

Rebuilding self-trust after heartbreak sets the stage for healthier relationships of all kinds, not just romantic ones. You will notice:

- **Better Friendships**: You choose friends who respect your boundaries and do not force you to second-guess yourself.
- **Improved Work Life**: Confidence in your judgment can lead to better performance, negotiations, or career choices.
- **Peace of Mind**: Instead of constant mental battles, you learn to back your own decisions, freeing up energy for growth and enjoyment of life.

---

19. Consistency Is Key

Self-trust, like muscle strength, improves through consistent exercises. You might do well for a few weeks and then have a setback. That is normal.

- **Plan for Slumps**: If you notice you are slipping back into old doubts, revisit the basics—journaling, affirmations, or small decision challenges.
- **Celebrate Comebacks**: Each time you realize you have lapsed and you correct course, that is evidence your new habits are taking root.

---

20. Conclusion of Chapter 9

Rebuilding trust in yourself is one of the most critical steps toward a healthier emotional future after heartbreak. By acknowledging your mistakes without condemning yourself, by practicing small decision-making exercises, and by gradually re-engaging with social and romantic scenarios, you reinforce the idea that your judgment is valid. You are not doomed to repeat your past errors. Instead, you can carry lessons from your previous heartbreak into a new era of self-confidence.

As you continue to heal, remember that self-trust is a skill—one that takes time, patience, and consistent practice. In the next chapter, we will look at learning from past experiences. We will examine how to understand patterns, break them, and create a more positive outlook on relationships. This next phase involves putting your new self-trust into action by analyzing past events with a clear mind and open heart.

Chapter 10: Learning from Past Experiences

After heartbreak, it is natural to replay memories of the relationship—sometimes on a loop. However, if replaying the past only stirs anger, shame, or regret, it can lead to getting stuck rather than growing. This chapter is about turning those memories into constructive lessons. You will discover how to examine past experiences in a fair, balanced manner, identify patterns that may have contributed to heartbreak, and build new ways of thinking that allow you to approach future relationships with more wisdom.

---

1. Why Reflecting on the Past Matters

Many people want to forget their old relationship entirely. The pain feels too raw. Yet, ignoring the past can lead you to repeat the same emotional cycles. Reflection is a way to transform painful memories into stepping stones toward healthier choices.

- **Identify Patterns**: You might see that you consistently choose partners who do not respect your boundaries, or that you tend to hide your real feelings until conflict explodes.
- **Gain Self-Awareness**: Reflection can show how your upbringing, your self-image, or your assumptions about love shaped your behavior.
- **Make Peace**: Proper reflection can reduce the power of guilt or anger by showing you a clearer picture of what really happened.

---

2. Signs You Are Ruminating Rather Than Learning

Rumination involves going over the same thoughts again and again, with no new insights. It keeps you trapped in bitterness or regret. **Learning** involves stepping back, gathering lessons, and deciding on actions for the future.

- **Rumination**: "I cannot believe they said that to me. I'm so dumb. I can't stop replaying that last argument."
- **Learning**: "They used that phrase, and I felt worthless. Next time, if someone speaks to me like that, I will walk away or address it calmly."

To shift from rumination to learning, start by noticing when your thoughts are circling without any productive outcome. Then, guide yourself toward a question: "What can I take from this to do better in the future?"

---

3. The Emotional Stages of Reflection

Reflecting on a breakup is not a neat process. Emotions can swing from sadness to anger to confusion. Recognizing these stages can help you be patient with yourself:

1. **Denial and Shock**: You might refuse to believe the relationship is over or that you played any part in problems.
2. **Anger**: You blame your ex or yourself, looking for someone to carry responsibility for the hurt.
3. **Sadness and Regret**: You mourn missed opportunities or realized flaws.
4. **Understanding**: Over time, you see the bigger picture. You can admit both sides had strengths and faults.
5. **Acceptance**: You begin to let go, seeing the breakup as an event that, while painful, can teach important lessons.

It is normal to move back and forth between these stages. Healing is rarely linear.

---

4. Methods for Meaningful Reflection

4.1. Structured Journaling

Use guided questions to analyze the past relationship:

- **What Drew You Together Initially?**: List qualities that attracted you to your ex or made the connection appealing. Were these qualities actually present, or were they what you hoped to see?
- **What Kept You Invested?**: Reflect on why you stayed, even if you noticed problems. Did fear, insecurity, or social pressure play a role?
- **What Broke Down Communication?**: Identify moments when either you or your ex shut down, argued unfairly, or let misunderstandings grow.

- **Positive Contributions**: Acknowledge the times you showed kindness, honesty, or tried to fix problems.
- **Lessons**: Write at least one lesson from each section of your journal. For example, "I learned that ignoring red flags does not make them vanish."

4.2. Timeline Approach

- **Chronological Steps**: On a piece of paper, write down key milestones of your relationship in order—first date, first big fight, major changes, final disagreement.
- **Note Shifts in Behavior**: Mark on the timeline where trust was lost or boundaries were crossed. This can help you see how small issues might have grown into bigger ones over time.

5. Identifying Repetitive Patterns

If this breakup was not your first, think about any repeating themes across past relationships:

- **Similar Personality Types**: Do you often choose partners who are emotionally unavailable, controlling, or distant?
- **Your Response Style**: Do you see a pattern where you avoid confrontation until it becomes explosive, or do you become overly accommodating?
- **Escalation Behaviors**: Look at how arguments typically escalated. Did you or your ex make them worse by bringing up past grudges or name-calling?

Seeing these patterns does not mean you are doomed to repeat them. Instead, awareness can help you break the cycle by making different choices next time.

6. Handling Guilt and Shame

When you realize how certain actions hurt the relationship, guilt or shame can creep in. Guilt can be a sign you recognize you did something wrong, which can be a catalyst for change. Shame, on the other hand, can make you believe you are a bad person at your core.

- **Separate Guilt from Identity**: If you lied or acted poorly, it does not mean you are forever dishonest or unworthy. It means you need to address that behavior and commit to not repeating it.
- **Apologize if Appropriate**: If it is safe and relevant, a sincere apology might ease your guilt. However, sometimes an apology is impossible or unwise—use your judgment.
- **Self-Forgiveness Practices**: Write a letter to yourself acknowledging what you did wrong and how you plan to change. Then read it when shame tries to overwhelm you.

7. Understanding the Other Person's Role

Learning from the past does not mean taking all the blame. A relationship involves two people. While you do not want to become stuck in blaming your ex for everything, it is still helpful to acknowledge their part in the breakdown.

- **Unfair Behaviors**: Did your ex lie, manipulate, or verbally attack you? Recognizing these behaviors helps you know what you will not tolerate next time.
- **Mutual Tensions**: Sometimes both sides contributed to negativity by refusing to communicate or by fueling each other's anger. Understanding this dynamic helps you see the role both parties played.
- **Own Only Your Share**: You cannot fix or change what your ex did, but you can focus on how you reacted and how you might handle it differently in the future.

8. Turning Lessons into Action Steps

Reflection is only as good as the changes it inspires. Once you know your patterns, plan concrete ways to act differently:

- **Boundary Setting**: If you discovered you allowed disrespect, commit to speaking up as soon as you sense it.
- **Communication Style**: If you realized you tend to withdraw in fights, practice being more direct. This might involve calmly stating, "I feel upset right now. Can we talk about this openly?"

- **Choosing Better Partners**: Make a list of red flags you will not overlook again, as well as green flags (positive traits) that suggest someone may be a healthier match.

---

9. Avoiding Extreme Reactions

Sometimes learning from heartbreak can push people to extremes:

- **Complete Emotional Shutdown**: Declaring you will never date again or trust anyone, ever. This reaction is understandable but can lead to isolation.
- **Rebound Relationships**: Jumping too quickly into a new relationship to prove you have learned something, or to distract from pain, often leads to more heartache.
- **Rigid Rules**: Creating a checklist so strict (e.g., "I will only date someone who texts me five times a day, never gets angry, shares all my interests") that no real person can qualify.

Balance is key. The goal is not to form an impenetrable wall but to find guidelines that protect your well-being while allowing genuine connection.

---

10. Seeking Outside Perspectives

Friends, counselors, or support groups can sometimes see your patterns more clearly than you can. Asking for feedback can strengthen your learning process.

- **Close Friends**: They might point out that you always seem to date people who do not value your career goals, or that you become too passive during conflicts.
- **Therapists**: Professionals can help you dig deeper, exploring past wounds or family beliefs that keep repeating in your adult relationships.
- **Mentors or Role Models**: If you know someone who has a healthy relationship, ask how they handle arguments, trust, or personal boundaries. Their experiences can guide you.

11. Letting Go of the "What Ifs"

Learning from the past does not mean agonizing over every potential alternative. "What if I had said something different?" "What if I had ended it sooner?" Overthinking like this can become a mental trap.

- **Acknowledge Past Realities**: You made the best decisions you could at the time, given your emotional state and the information you had.
- **Focus on the Present**: Each "what if" question can be turned into an action plan for the future: "Next time I see that pattern, I will leave earlier" or "Next time I sense I'm unhappy, I will speak up sooner."

---

12. Applying Lessons Beyond Romance

The insights you gain from heartbreak can apply to friendships, family dynamics, and professional settings. For instance:

- **Boundary Lessons**: If you learned the importance of setting limits in romantic relationships, you can use that knowledge to handle a pushy coworker or a demanding family member.
- **Emotional Regulation**: If you discovered you tend to lash out when stressed, you can apply self-soothing methods at work or in other social interactions.
- **Communication Upgrades**: Improved communication skills—like stating your needs clearly and listening without interrupting—are valuable in any close relationship.

---

13. Celebrating (Acknowledging) Growth Milestones

- **Track Progress**: Keep a small journal or note on your phone about lessons you have learned and how you apply them. Write down each time you handle a situation in a healthier way than before.
- **Share with Trusted Allies**: It can be motivating to tell a friend, "I recognized a red flag and spoke up instead of ignoring it. I'm proud of this step."

- **Reward Yourself**: After making a significant improvement—like calmly resolving an argument—treat yourself to something small you enjoy, such as a relaxing walk in nature or a favorite snack.

---

14. Handling Relapses or Emotional Setbacks

You might find yourself repeating an old pattern despite your best intentions. For example, you might stay silent during a conflict until resentment builds. This does not erase all your progress.

- **Identify the Trigger**: Try to figure out what caused the old behavior. Were you tired, stressed, or afraid of conflict?
- **Practice Self-Forgiveness**: Say something like, "I slipped up, but I am still learning."
- **Plan a Correction**: Next time, you might decide, "I will speak up as soon as I notice I'm feeling uneasy, rather than waiting."

---

15. Visualizing Positive Relationship Scenarios

While heartbreak can leave you with negative memories, imagining a healthier connection can help shift your mindset:

- **Envision Future Interactions**: Picture yourself in a balanced relationship where you communicate openly, respect each other's needs, and handle disagreements with maturity.
- **Feel the Emotions**: Focus on the emotions you would have—calmness, security, mutual respect—rather than dwelling on fear of repeating the past.
- **Use This Vision as a Guide**: When meeting new people, compare your real experiences to your vision. Are they offering some of the traits you imagined, such as open communication and respect?

---

16. Creating a Personal Growth Plan

Sometimes it helps to formalize what you want to change, learn, or explore after heartbreak:

1. **Self-Knowledge Goals**
   - Aim to discover more about yourself, such as how you react under stress or what you truly value in a partner.
2. **Emotional Skills Goals**
   - Improve your ability to calm yourself during conflict, listen actively, or express your feelings with clarity.
3. **Boundary Goals**
   - Practice setting one new boundary each week, whether at work, with friends, or in casual dating.

Writing down these goals can make them feel more real and keep you accountable.

---

17. Recognizing When to Stop Digging

Though reflection is helpful, there can come a point where analyzing the past starts to harm your present. If you find yourself feeling depressed or anxious after every reflection session, it might be time to reduce or pause that process.

- **Time-Boxing Reflection**: Set a limit (e.g., 20 minutes) for daily reflection, and then engage in an uplifting activity.
- **Seek Professional Help**: If reflection triggers severe emotional pain or you cannot move past certain memories, a counselor can guide you through deeper healing in a structured way.

---

18. The Upside of Past Heartbreak

It might sound strange, but heartbreak can lead to growth that you might not have achieved otherwise. Sometimes it pushes you to question assumptions, develop assertiveness, or identify patterns that needed to change. People often say they feel more self-aware and more certain about what they want after a tough breakup.

- **Resilience Building**: Overcoming heartbreak can teach you that you can survive deep pain and emerge stronger.
- **Clearer Goals**: You might realize you want a partner who shares certain values or life ambitions, whereas before you had not thought carefully about it.

- **Better Self-Esteem**: As you learn from mistakes and see your growth, you gain confidence in your ability to handle challenges.

19. Sharing Your Lessons Responsibly

You might be eager to tell others what you have learned, especially if they are also going through heartbreak. Sharing experiences can be a good thing, but be mindful:

- **Offer, Don't Preach**: Share your insights as suggestions, not commands. "This helped me," not "You must do this."
- **Respect Boundaries**: Some people are not ready to hear advice. They may just need a listening ear.
- **Balance Vulnerability**: While being open can bond people, do not feel obligated to share every detail of your heartbreak with casual acquaintances.

20. Conclusion of Chapter 10

Learning from past experiences is an active process. It involves sifting through memories, identifying useful lessons, and applying them in daily life. Instead of running from the pain of heartbreak, you can choose to transform that pain into something constructive. Through reflection, you identify patterns, correct harmful behaviors, and set healthier boundaries. By doing so, you lay a solid foundation for better relationships in the future—both romantic and otherwise.

Remember that true learning does not happen all at once. It unfolds over time as you notice old triggers and apply new behaviors. You may have setbacks, but each setback can itself be part of your ongoing education in self-awareness and emotional maturity. In the following chapters, we will continue exploring how to build confidence, communicate effectively, and move forward with renewed strength. You do not have to forget your past heartbreak; you can use it as fuel to create a life that feels more aligned with who you truly want to be.

Chapter 11: Confidence-Building Practices

After heartbreak, your sense of worth and capability may feel shaken. You might question whether you are good enough in your personal life, professional life, or simply as a human being. This chapter will explore concrete ways to build confidence and a strong sense of self, even when emotional wounds are fresh. While heartbreak can leave you feeling uncertain, it also creates space to form new habits and mindsets that reinforce a solid self-image.

---

1. Defining Confidence

Confidence is the belief that you can handle challenges, learn from mistakes, and present yourself without fear of constant judgment. It does not mean bragging or thinking you are flawless. Rather, it allows you to trust that you have something of value to offer, whether it is in friendships, at work, or in personal pursuits.

- **Not Arrogance**: Confidence does not require you to look down on others or pretend to be superior.
- **Adaptable**: Confidence can grow or diminish depending on life events. A major heartbreak might lower your self-esteem temporarily, but it can recover.
- **Internal vs. External**: True confidence comes from within. Though external achievements help, it is the inner sense of worth that keeps you steady.

---

2. Why Heartbreak Shakes Confidence

1. **Emotional Distress**
    - When a relationship ends, it can feel like a personal failure. You might question what you did wrong or why you "couldn't make it work."
    - This distress can sap your motivation to pursue hobbies, friendships, or career goals.
2. **Loss of External Validation**

- If your partner once provided regular compliments or support, their absence can leave a void.
- You might have leaned on their words to feel good about yourself. Without them, you might feel insecure.

3. **Self-Doubt**
    - You could worry that you misread signals or ignored negative behaviors. This might make you think, "If I was wrong about this, maybe I am wrong about other things."
    - It becomes easy to second-guess your instincts or decisions.

---

3. Building Confidence from the Inside Out

3.1. Acknowledge What You Already Do Well

- **List Your Strengths**: Write down five to ten things you are good at or character traits you are proud of, such as being empathetic, resourceful, good at organizing, or funny.
- **Ask Trusted Friends**: Sometimes others can see your strengths more clearly. Let them share positive qualities they see in you.

3.2. Tackle Small Goals First

- **Pick One Simple Objective**: Maybe it is organizing a section of your closet or learning a new recipe. Achieving small tasks can create a sense of competence.
- **Celebrate Internally**: When you complete a goal, allow yourself a quiet moment of recognition: "I did that. I am capable."

3.3. Observe Self-Talk

- **Replace "I Can't"**: Each time you catch yourself saying, "I can't handle this," or "I'm not good enough," pause. Then try to reframe: "I'm learning to handle this," or "I have resources to improve."
- **Speak as a Supportive Friend**: If a close friend were in your shoes, you would likely offer kind words. Practice giving that same compassion to yourself.

---

4. Physical Activities That Boost Confidence

Our bodies and minds are linked, so activities that engage your body can affect your mental self-image.

4.1. Posture Awareness

- **Stand Tall**: Align your back and shoulders, allowing your chest to open and your head to remain level. This posture can reduce feelings of shame or timidity.
- **Breathing Exercises**: Inhale slowly while counting to four, hold briefly, then exhale for a count of four. Steady breaths calm the mind, reinforcing a sense of stability.

4.2. Movement or Exercise

- **Moderate Workouts**: Something as simple as a daily walk, short stretching routine, or home workout session can release mood-lifting endorphins.
- **Mind-Body Practices**: Some people find that calm, meditative styles of movement (like light yoga-type routines) improve body awareness and thus self-confidence.
- **Tracking Progress**: Keep a small log of your workouts or steps per day. Watching your strength or stamina grow can translate into feeling more self-assured overall.

4.3. Dress in a Way That Lifts Your Mood

- **Comfort and Style**: You do not have to wear expensive clothes, but choosing outfits that make you feel comfortable and presentable can shift your mental state.
- **Small Acts of Grooming**: Taking the time to fix your hair, do simple skin care, or wear something that makes you feel put together can boost how you see yourself.

---

5. Challenging Negative Beliefs

After heartbreak, it is easy to fall into the trap of harmful beliefs like "I am unlovable" or "I will always fail."

5.1. Thought Record Approach

- **Identify the Belief**: For example, "I am unlovable."
- **Look for Evidence**: Ask yourself, "Is this 100% true? Have there been times someone valued me?"
- **Replace with Balanced Thought**: Something like, "One relationship ended, but that does not mean I am forever unlovable."

5.2. Stop Comparing

- **Cut Down Social Media**: Limit time spent looking at others' highlight reels, which can feed jealousy or a sense of inadequacy.
- **Focus on Your Path**: Remind yourself that your growth and timeline are unique. Another person's apparent success or happiness does not diminish your worth.

---

6. Developing Skills for Personal Growth

Learning new skills or improving existing talents can dramatically increase your confidence. It provides a sense of progress and control over your life.

6.1. Pick an Interest That Excites You

- **Hobbies**: This can be anything from painting, coding, baking, to learning a musical instrument. A new hobby can bring a refreshing focus outside the heartbreak.
- **Online Courses or Tutorials**: With today's resources, you can find beginner-friendly classes on nearly any topic, often for free or low cost.
- **Celebrate (Acknowledge) Milestones**: Each time you finish a course module or successfully create something new, note it as a sign of your evolving capabilities.

6.2. Professional Development

- **Career Goals**: If you feel uncertain in your personal life, focusing on work or career development can give structure. Setting a goal like applying for a new position or taking a certification course can boost self-assurance.
- **Mentorship**: Seek out a mentor or a supportive colleague who can guide your professional growth.

7. Building Supportive Connections

Confidence can grow when you have people around who encourage your strengths and respect your feelings.

7.1. Positive Friendships

- **Quality over Quantity**: A few close friends who genuinely care about you can be more uplifting than a large circle of superficial acquaintances.
- **Mutual Respect**: Look for friends who listen without constant judgment, and make sure you return the favor.

7.2. Networking with Like-Minded Individuals

- **Groups or Clubs**: Joining local or online groups dedicated to your interests can help you find a supportive community.
- **Sharing Skills**: Offering your knowledge or support within a group can remind you of your value.

8. Handling Setbacks and Doubt

Confidence-building is not a straight line. You might feel strong one day and then have a setback. This is normal.

8.1. Plan for Low Days

- **Self-Soothing Techniques**: Keep a list of soothing actions, like a warm bath, a brief walk, or listening to a calm playlist.
- **Affirmation Cards**: Write some encouraging phrases on small cards. Read them when negativity creeps in.

8.2. Recognize Progress

- **Track It**: Use a notebook or an app where you write down each small success—finishing a project, speaking up in a meeting, or resisting negative self-talk.
- **Reward System**: After hitting certain milestones, treat yourself in a simple way, like cooking a nice meal or visiting a local park.

9. Speaking Up for Yourself

Confidence is often displayed through the way you communicate. If you tend to keep your thoughts hidden, practicing open expression can boost your self-belief.

9.1. Begin with Minor Disagreements

- **Practice in Safe Spaces**: If a friend says something you disagree with, calmly share your viewpoint rather than staying silent.
- **Respectful Tone**: Being direct does not mean being rude. Aim for clear, firm statements without insults or raised voices.

9.2. Express Needs in Personal Relationships

- **Set Boundaries**: If someone is pushing you past your comfort zone, politely but firmly say what you need. "I'm not comfortable discussing that topic," or "I need some space right now."
- **Ask for What You Want**: Instead of hoping people will guess, plainly say: "It would help me if you could..." or "I would like more time to talk about this."

---

10. Unconventional Confidence-Boosting Methods

Here are a few less common ideas that can yield surprising results:

1. **Power Poses**
   - Some research suggests that standing in an open, confident pose (e.g., hands on hips, shoulders back) for a minute can temporarily raise feelings of empowerment.
   - Do this in private if you feel self-conscious. It can help you mentally shift before a challenging task.
2. **Volunteering**
   - Helping others can remind you that you have skills and compassion to offer. Whether it is reading to children, assisting at a shelter, or walking dogs at a rescue, purposeful acts can raise your self-worth.
3. **Recording Voice Notes**
   - Many people find writing journals to be useful, but if you prefer speaking, record short messages to yourself about what you did

well that day or what you want to improve. Hearing your own voice reaffirm your strengths can be powerful.
   4. **Daily Micro-Challenges**
      - Challenge yourself to do one small, slightly uncomfortable thing per day—like talking to a stranger in line or trying a new recipe. Over time, these micro-challenges stretch your comfort zone and boost confidence.

---

11. Overcoming Fear of Criticism

One reason heartbreak can crush confidence is the fear of future rejection or judgment. Handling criticism in a healthier way can help you step forward with more certainty.

- **Constructive vs. Harsh Criticism**: If someone gives you valid tips on how to improve, that can be helpful. If they insult you without clear reasons, that is their negativity, not necessarily your truth.
- **Responding Calmly**: Instead of reacting defensively, pause. Ask yourself if there is any merit in the criticism. If yes, note it. If no, let it go.
- **Self-Acceptance**: Recognize that you cannot please everyone. Having your own values and goals means some people will disagree.

---

12. Translating Confidence into New Opportunities

As your confidence grows, you might notice more chances for a fulfilling life:

1. **Social Invitations**
   - You could feel more comfortable attending events or gatherings, leading to new friendships or professional connections.
2. **Career Steps**
   - Confidence might drive you to apply for a promotion, change jobs, or start your own small venture.
3. **Personal Adventures**
   - You may decide to travel somewhere close by (for a weekend) or join a local class you once felt too shy to try. Feeling more self-assured paves the way for broader experiences.

13. Balancing Confidence with Humility

It is important to keep confidence from turning into arrogance. True confidence does not require showing off or insisting you are always right.

- **Admit Mistakes**: If you realize you were wrong, say so. Acknowledging errors can show that you are secure enough not to hide flaws.
- **Stay Curious**: Being open to learning suggests that you respect your own capabilities while recognizing there is always more to understand.
- **Support Others**: Confident people often enjoy lifting others up because they do not fear losing their place.

---

14. Avoiding Overreliance on External Validation

Sometimes a new love interest, social media likes, or compliments from coworkers can temporarily boost your sense of self. While these are pleasant, relying on them too heavily can be risky.

- **Internal Metrics**: Focus on your progress, values, and self-assessment to measure your worth.
- **Self-Appraisal**: After doing a task, ask yourself, "Did I handle that in line with my standards and potential?" rather than waiting for others to praise you.

---

15. The Link Between Confidence and Emotional Health

When you work on feeling stronger about who you are, it becomes easier to manage emotions like sadness, anger, or loneliness. You trust your resilience.

- **Less Anxiety**: You worry less about every possibility because you believe you can handle the outcomes.
- **Better Emotional Regulation**: Confidence can stabilize your mood, especially when faced with unexpected changes or conflicts.
- **Healthier Relationships**: Partners or friends often respect someone who values themselves. They see that you will not tolerate unhealthy behavior, and this sets a positive tone.

16. Checking In with Yourself Regularly

Confidence is not a one-time achievement. It is like a skill you strengthen through ongoing practice.

1. **Weekly Review**
   - Take a few minutes to think about areas where you felt proud or where you allowed fear to silence you.
2. **Note Patterns**
   - Do you lose confidence in social settings, work meetings, or romantic conversations? Recognizing these triggers can help you prepare next time.
3. **Adjust Tactics**
   - If something did not work (like a certain affirmation or a certain approach to boundary-setting), change it and try again.

---

17. Healing Childhood Roots of Low Confidence

Some women discover that heartbreak taps into earlier self-esteem issues, possibly from critical parents or bullying experiences. Addressing these deeper roots can bring lasting change.

- **Therapy or Counseling**: A professional can help you untangle old narratives about your worth.
- **Inner Child Exercises**: Techniques where you offer kindness and reassurance to the younger version of yourself can aid healing.
- **Support Groups**: Sharing experiences with those who faced similar childhood challenges can help normalize your feelings.

---

18. Watching Out for Self-Sabotage

Sometimes, as you start feeling better about yourself, old habits or fears might tempt you to sabotage your progress. You might pick fights, procrastinate on goals, or dismiss compliments.

- **Recognize Self-Sabotage Signs**: You suddenly lose interest in a project you used to care about, or you push away supportive friends.

- **Pause and Reflect**: Ask, "Why am I undermining my own progress?" Often, it is fear of failing or being hurt again.
- **Create Accountability**: Ask a friend or mentor to check in with you if they notice you slipping back into negative patterns.

---

19. Celebrating (Acknowledging) Ongoing Succes

- **Visible Markers**: Place reminders around your room of how far you have come, such as notes about past achievements.
- **Social Sharing**: If you feel comfortable, share a success story with a supportive friend or group. Feedback can reinforce your sense of progress.
- **Revisit Before-and-After Mindsets**: Compare your current thoughts to how you felt right after the breakup. Notice the shift in your approach to life.

---

20. Conclusion of Chapter 11

Confidence is not a magical trait reserved for certain people—it is a set of practices and mindsets you can develop, especially after heartbreak. By tuning into your strengths, challenging negative beliefs, and taking steady steps forward, you can create a lasting sense of self-assuredness. This does not mean you will never have bad days or feel unsure; it means you will bounce back from those moments more quickly.

Your increased confidence can enhance every part of your life, from your friendships to your career choices to any future romances. Self-belief allows you to walk boldly, knowing that you have something valuable to share with the world. In the next chapter, we will explore communication tips that can help you build healthier connections. Confidence feeds directly into clear, respectful communication—a key skill for any future relationship or meaningful bond.

Chapter 12: Communication Tips for Future Relationships

Good communication forms the backbone of any healthy relationship. After a heartbreak, you might be wary of opening up or might fear repeating past conflicts. This chapter will guide you through effective communication methods, showing you how to speak your thoughts in a way that fosters mutual respect. Whether you are looking ahead to a new romantic connection or hoping to improve relationships with friends and family, these strategies can help you form deeper, more authentic bonds.

---

1. Why Communication Matters After Heartbreak

1. **Misunderstandings Led to Pain**
   - In many breakups, poor communication—like failing to express needs or not hearing the other person's viewpoint—plays a big role.
   - Learning better communication can reduce the likelihood of similar issues recurring.
2. **Trust and Openness**
   - If trust was broken, you may be wary of expressing your real feelings. However, honest discussion is key for rebuilding trust in your future connections.
3. **Emotional Healing**
   - Verbalizing what you went through can help you release emotional burdens. It also allows new partners or close friends to understand your perspective.

---

2. Identifying Your Communication Style

We all have default tendencies in how we express ourselves. Understanding your style can help you refine it.

- **Passive**: Avoiding stating opinions or feelings openly. Often leads to pent-up resentment or confusion.

- **Aggressive**: Communicating in a demanding or insulting way. Can cause fear or defensiveness in others.
- **Passive-Aggressive**: Indirectly expressing anger or frustration, such as giving silent treatment or sarcastic remarks. This approach avoids direct confrontation but breeds tension.
- **Assertive**: Respectfully and clearly stating one's thoughts, while honoring the other person's feelings. This is generally the healthiest style.

3. The Basics of Assertive Communication

Assertiveness helps you speak honestly without bulldozing the other person.

1. **Use "I" Statements**
   - Instead of saying "You never listen," say, "I feel ignored when I try to share something and you look at your phone."
   - This lowers defensiveness and focuses on your feelings rather than blaming the other person.
2. **Specific Feedback**
   - Vague complaints like "You are mean" are not helpful. Stating specifics—"I feel upset when you interrupt me during disagreements"—is clearer and more likely to lead to change.
3. **Stay Calm**
   - Yelling or cursing often results in the other person shutting down. If you feel anger rising, try deep breaths or a short break.
4. **Ask for Their Perspective**
   - Assertive communication is not one-sided. Invite the other person to explain their thoughts: "Can you share how you feel about this situation?"

4. Listening Skills

Communication is not just about talking. It also involves truly hearing what the other person says.

4.1. Active Listening

- **Eye Contact**: Put aside distractions like phones. Show that you are fully present.

- **Reflective Responses**: Summarize what the speaker said in your own words to confirm understanding. For example, "So you feel hurt because I was late?"
- **No Interruptions**: Let the other person finish speaking before you reply. This helps them feel heard and reduces tension.

4.2. Empathy

- **Imagine Their Point of View**: Even if you disagree, try to see where they are coming from. This can lower hostility.
- **Validate Feelings**: You do not have to agree with their conclusions, but you can acknowledge their emotions. "I see this makes you upset."

---

5. Overcoming Fear of Speaking Up

If your last relationship ended badly, you may be afraid to raise concerns in new interactions. You might think, "What if I scare them away?" or "What if they reject me for speaking honestly?"

1. **Gradual Practice**
   - Begin by voicing small preferences, like which restaurant you prefer. Build up to bigger topics.
2. **Fear-Setting Exercise**
   - Ask yourself: "What is the worst thing that could happen if I express this thought?" Often, the outcome is less dire than you imagine.
3. **Recognize Your Rights**
   - You have the right to your opinions, needs, and emotions. A person who cannot handle them may not be a suitable friend or partner.

---

6. Communicating Boundaries

Post-heartbreak, you might want to set clearer boundaries to avoid past mistakes. This may involve what you will tolerate, how often you need alone time, or how you handle disagreements.

6.1. Define Them First

- **Know Your Limits**: You cannot communicate boundaries unless you are clear on them yourself. For example, "I am not okay with shouting or name-calling," or "I need a day to myself each week."

6.2. State Them Plainly

- **Short and Clear**: "I need us to speak without raising our voices." Overly long explanations can muddle the main point.
- **Explain Why (If Helpful)**: "When you shout, I feel scared and shut down. I respond better if we speak calmly."

6.3. Be Consistent

- **Follow Through**: If the boundary is crossed, address it immediately. Letting it slide sends the message that you do not really mean it.
- **Fair Enforcement**: Boundaries apply to you as well. If you expect calm talking, you should also avoid yelling.

---

7. Handling Conflict Respectfully

Conflicts are normal in any connection. The key is managing them in a way that promotes resolution instead of causing deeper rifts.

7.1. "Time-Out" Method

- **Pause**: If emotions run high, either person can request a short break: "I need ten minutes to calm down before continuing."
- **Return to Discussion**: Ensure you come back to the topic rather than using breaks to dodge the issue entirely.

7.2. Problem-Solving Approach

- **Identify the Core Issue**: Often, the fight is not about the surface complaint. Maybe it is about feeling unappreciated or stressed at work.
- **Brainstorm Solutions**: Work together to find ways to address the root of the conflict.
- **Agree on a Plan**: Even if neither of you gets everything you want, a partial solution can maintain mutual respect.

8. Addressing Past Trauma or Hurt

If your previous heartbreak involved deception, emotional mistreatment, or other trauma, discussing this with a new partner can be daunting. However, sharing relevant parts of your history can help them understand you better.

1. **Share Gradually**
   - You do not have to reveal everything on the first date or conversation. Wait until you feel some trust has been established.
2. **Explain Triggers**
   - If certain actions or words trigger intense reactions because of past wounds, let your new partner know. This allows them to be more mindful.
3. **Clarify What You Need**
   - For example, "I need reassurance sometimes because I was lied to in my previous relationship." This is not begging for sympathy—rather, it is giving them tools to better connect with you.

9. Nonverbal Communication

Words are only one part of interaction. Facial expressions, gestures, and tone of voice can reveal or hide a great deal.

- **Maintain Appropriate Eye Contact**: Looking away constantly can signal disinterest or hiding. Staring too intensely might be off-putting.
- **Be Mindful of Your Tone**: The same words can sound supportive or sarcastic depending on how you say them.
- **Respect Personal Space**: Notice if the other person seems uncomfortable with your proximity. Likewise, if you need more space, express that.

10. Digital Communication Tips

In modern life, texting and social media often replace face-to-face interaction. While convenient, they can lead to misunderstandings.

10.1. Clarity in Texts

- **Use Calm Language**: Sarcasm or jokes do not always come across well in text. Add clarifications if needed.
- **Avoid Long, Heated Messages**: If upset, consider a phone call or an in-person talk. Text rants can spiral and be misread.

10.2. Social Media Boundaries

- **Privacy Settings**: Decide how much of your personal life (and potential new relationship) you want to share online.
- **Conflict Offline**: If a disagreement arises, handle it privately. Public posts can escalate drama.
- **Stop Monitoring**: Avoid the urge to constantly check an ex's profile or to compare your new partner's online activity with your ex's behavior.

---

11. Communicating in New Romantic Encounters

If you decide to date again, strong communication from the start can set the tone.

- **State Intentions**: If you want a serious relationship, say so early on. If you are just exploring options, be honest.
- **Discuss Relationship Values**: Talk about what matters to you—honesty, respect, time together, independence, etc.—and ask them about their values.
- **Gradual Disclosure**: Reveal personal details at a pace that feels comfortable for both sides.

---

12. Handling Rejection or Disinterest

Healthy communication includes how you respond if a connection does not work out.

- **Stay Civil**: Name-calling or blaming only intensifies hurt feelings. If someone is not interested, that is their right.
- **Acknowledge Feelings**: It is okay to say you feel disappointed or sad. This honesty is more mature than pretending you do not care.

- **Part on Mutual Respect**: If possible, end conversations or relationships on a note that respects both parties' dignity.

13. Communication in Friendships Post-Heartbreak

Your approach to communication also affects friends. Maybe they feel uncertain about how to talk to you, or you have changed your priorities and schedules.

1. **Check-In Chats**
   - Let your friends know what you need. A simple "I appreciate you checking on me, but I might not always want to talk about the breakup" can clarify boundaries.
2. **Be Direct About New Preferences**
   - If you are trying to avoid certain events (e.g., seeing your ex), let friends know in advance so they can plan accordingly.

14. Repairing Communication with Family

If heartbreak affected family relationships—maybe they disapproved of your ex or criticized you—open communication can clear the air.

- **Acknowledgment**: If they said something hurtful, calmly point it out: "It hurt me when you kept saying I was at fault."
- **Mutual Understanding**: Ask them to share their concerns. Understanding their viewpoint can reduce tension.
- **Seek Mediation**: If the situation is tense, a family counselor can moderate a conversation where everyone feels heard.

15. Maintaining Healthy Dialogue Long-Term

Effective communication is not a one-time fix; it requires consistent effort.

1. **Schedule Regular Talks**
   - In a new relationship, set aside time—maybe weekly—to discuss how each person feels, any concerns, or updates.

2. **Revisit Boundaries**
   - Boundaries may evolve as the relationship grows. Keep each other updated if something changes.
3. **Address Small Issues Early**
   - Do not wait for frustrations to accumulate. Tackle them while they are still minor annoyances.

---

16. Avoiding Over-Sharing

While honesty is key, dumping every single detail or fear on someone can be overwhelming—especially early in a relationship or friendship.

- **Pace Yourself**: Share relevant information that helps the bond grow, but let the relationship develop before revealing very personal or heavy issues.
- **Gauge Reactions**: Notice if the other person seems comfortable or if they are pulling back. Adjust how much you share accordingly.

---

17. Teaching Others How You Wish to Be Treated

By consistently communicating your boundaries, needs, and feelings, you teach others what treatment you accept or refuse.

- **Lead by Example**: If you expect respect, show respect. If you wish for honesty, be honest in return.
- **Consistency**: The more consistent you are, the clearer your message. If you sometimes let people disrespect you, they get mixed signals.

---

18. Warning Signs of Unhealthy Communication

Even if you use healthy methods, sometimes the other person responds poorly. Recognizing red flags can help you decide whether the connection is worth saving.

- **Frequent Name-Calling or Yelling**: Occasional anger is normal, but persistent verbal attacks signal deeper issues.

- **Gaslighting**: When someone denies your reality or manipulates you into questioning your sanity, it is a major red flag.
- **Chronic Stonewalling**: If the other person repeatedly refuses to talk or vanishes whenever a serious topic arises, it can block any chance of resolution.

---

19. Seeking Help When Needed

In some relationships—romantic or otherwise—communication problems may be entrenched. You might need external support to resolve them.

- **Couples Counseling**: If you and a new partner face misunderstandings but want to fix them, therapy can provide tools and a neutral space.
- **Conflict Mediation**: For family feuds or roommate disputes, a mediator might help keep discussions on track.
- **Personal Therapy**: If you find yourself repeating communication mistakes, a counselor can help you identify triggers and work on new habits.

---

20. Conclusion of Chapter 12

Good communication is crucial for rebuilding trust and forming healthier relationships after heartbreak. It involves expressing your needs confidently and listening with empathy. While this can be challenging—especially if your previous connection ended in conflict—practicing assertive speaking, clear boundaries, and active listening can transform how you relate to others.

Whether you are opening up to a potential partner, talking with friends, or addressing family issues, strong communication reduces misinterpretation and fosters connection. It also sets a solid foundation for respect and mutual understanding. In the following chapters, we will explore how to handle single life after heartbreak, manage social pressures, and build a future that supports your emotional well-being. Keep these communication skills in mind as you navigate new possibilities, ensuring you maintain clarity and self-respect in all interactions.

Chapter 13: Handling Single Life After Heartbreak

When a romantic relationship ends, you may find yourself suddenly single. This can feel both freeing and deeply unsettling. For some women, it seems like the whole world is unfamiliar without the partner they grew used to. Others might feel relief if the relationship was stressful or harmful, but still experience moments of loneliness. This chapter aims to help you navigate the period of being single after heartbreak, offering ideas for emotional growth, practical tips for daily living, and uncommon insights to make this time more meaningful.

---

1. Understanding the Emotional Gap

After a breakup, a sense of emptiness can appear. You might have spent much of your time thinking about the relationship, planning things together, and sharing day-to-day routines. Suddenly, that closeness vanishes, leaving a space that feels strange.

- **Initial Turmoil**: The first few weeks can be rocky. Mood swings are common: one day you feel hopeful; the next you might feel lost.
- **Settling Period**: Eventually, a new rhythm can form. You begin to sleep and eat in a way that suits you, without worrying about someone else's schedule.
- **Redefining Yourself**: A single person's identity can be different from that of a person in a relationship. This shift can bring anxiety, but it can also bring fresh possibilities.

Uncommon Insight: Some mental health experts suggest taking a short online break at the beginning of single life—24 or 48 hours—just to reconnect with yourself without external influences. Turning off your phone and not checking social media can help you reflect on your own feelings and goals without constant noise from the outside world.

---

2. The Benefits of Single Life

Being single has real advantages. It might not always feel that way when you're grappling with heartbreak, but the single period can be a time of personal development that you might not get while in a busy or demanding relationship.

- **Freedom to Explore**: You can try new hobbies, adopt new routines, or take on challenges that you set aside during the relationship.
- **Deeper Friendships**: Sometimes, people devote most of their energy to a romantic partner and neglect friends. Being single can let you rebuild or strengthen friendships.
- **Personal Goals**: Career ambitions, creative projects, or travel (even a local road trip) can take center stage without having to negotiate your schedule with a partner.

Uncommon Insight: Some psychologists suggest you record a short audio each day—speaking your reflections, ideas, or feelings about what you did or learned. Over a few weeks, you can listen back and see how you're evolving. This is like an audio diary that captures your real-time growth during single life.

---

3. The Challenge of Loneliness

Though single life has benefits, loneliness can be a big hurdle, especially if you were used to sharing physical or emotional closeness.

1. **Recognize the Feeling**: Admit that you feel lonely. Loneliness is an emotional signal that your social or emotional needs aren't being fully met.
2. **Reach Out Wisely**: Instead of jumping into any new relationship right away, consider reaching out to friends, family, or social groups where you can feel supported without the pressure of romance.
3. **Healthy Distractions**: Activities like volunteering or attending small gatherings (in person or virtual) can offer social contact. The idea is not to avoid your sadness but to find positive ways to fill extra time.

Uncommon Insight: Research shows that certain forms of touch, even self-applied, can reduce feelings of loneliness. For example, placing a warm hand over your heart, or giving yourself a gentle shoulder rub, can activate parts of the brain associated with comfort. It sounds simple, but it can have a calming effect in moments of deep loneliness.

4. Reconnecting with Yourself

After heartbreak, your identity can feel shaky, as if part of you was defined by the relationship. Reconnecting with who you are independently can bring a sense of self-reliance.

- **List Personal Values**: Ask yourself what principles matter most to you: honesty, kindness, creativity, or freedom, for example. You might discover new aspects of yourself, or remember values you put aside.
- **Experiment with Hobbies**: Try different activities—maybe baking bread, playing a new instrument, or painting. You don't have to be "good" at them; exploration is enough.
- **Create a Personal Ritual**: Set aside a particular time each day for self-reflection: this could be writing in a journal, going for a short walk, or doing a 10-minute breathing exercise.

Uncommon Insight: Some coaches advise creating a "micro-room" in your home—one corner specifically designed for your favorite activity. Even if you only have a small apartment, designating a special corner for reading, writing, or crafting can give your mind a positive space to explore who you are without the influences of your past relationship.

---

5. Building Practical Routines

Being single can mean a change in daily structure. Maybe you used to share meals or plan weekends together. Now, you set your schedule. This can be intimidating but also liberating.

1. **Meal Planning**: Some people forget to eat well when they no longer cook for two. Writing a simple meal plan or trying new recipes can bring excitement and better nutrition.
2. **Sleep Habits**: Without a partner's bedtime routine, you might discover your best sleep schedule. Pay attention to how much rest makes you feel energized.
3. **Budgeting and Financial Steps**: If you shared finances with your ex or split bills, learn to manage your budget on your own. This might feel stressful at first, but financial independence often boosts confidence.

Uncommon Insight: Create a weekly mini-contract with yourself. For example, promise that "Monday, Wednesday, and Friday, I'll cook at home," or "Every evening by 10 p.m., I'll be away from my phone." Write it down, sign it, and post it somewhere visible. Treat it as an agreement with yourself, not just a casual idea.

---

6. Avoiding the Rebound Trap

A rebound relationship happens when someone starts a new romance quickly after a breakup, often to distract themselves from the pain of heartbreak. While it can provide short-term comfort, it rarely solves the deeper emotional issues.

- **Recognize Your Motives**: If you feel an intense urge to date right away, ask yourself if it's to fill a void or to genuinely explore a new connection.
- **Focus on Emotional Healing**: Give yourself time to process the breakup. Jumping from heartbreak to another relationship can lead to carrying old wounds into a new situation.
- **Talk to Trusted Friends**: Share your worries or excitement about a new crush with friends who know your breakup story. They might notice red flags or caution you if you're moving too fast.

Uncommon Insight: A helpful exercise is to write an "emotional readiness checklist." Include items like "I have processed my sadness in a healthy way," or "I feel strong enough to handle possible rejection." Check these off over a few weeks to track whether you're truly ready to start something new.

---

7. Expanding Your Social World

It's common to lose touch with certain friends during a relationship. Being single can open the door to reconnecting with old friends or forming new ones.

1. **Attend Group Activities**: Join a fitness class, a book club, or an arts workshop. Consistent gatherings allow you to meet people with similar interests.
2. **Online Communities**: If in-person meetings aren't possible or comfortable, find online groups related to your hobbies or professional field.
3. **Offer Help**: Volunteering for community projects can introduce you to kind-hearted people who also share a sense of purpose.

Uncommon Insight: Some cities host "silent meetups," where participants gather but communicate through notes or minimal speech to reduce social anxiety. If you're shy about meeting new people, see if something like this exists in your area or start your own low-pressure social event.

---

8. Traveling (Even Locally) as a Single Person

Traveling alone can be a powerful experience after heartbreak. While major trips might be expensive, even short local trips or day adventures can offer perspective.

- **Local Exploration**: Visit nearby towns or parks you've never seen. Exploring a new location alone can build confidence.
- **Travel Groups for Solo Women**: Some companies host tours specifically for single women. This can provide both safety and connection with others in a similar phase of life.
- **Document the Experience**: Take pictures or keep a mini travel journal. Reflecting later on your solo excursions can remind you of your independence.

Uncommon Insight: When traveling alone, try the "question jar method." Write down interesting questions about life or personal goals on small pieces of paper, place them in a jar, and bring them with you. Each day of your trip, draw one question and spend time pondering or writing about it. This can turn your travel into a deeper self-exploration activity.

---

9. Handling Pressure from People Around You

Friends, family, or coworkers might ask: "Are you dating yet?" or "When will you move on?" This can add stress.

- **Direct Communication**: Politely tell people that you're focusing on personal growth right now and are not rushing into dating.
- **Humor**: Sometimes a light-hearted remark can defuse nosy questions. "I'm too busy being fabulous on my own," for instance, can end a prying query.
- **Selective Sharing**: You don't owe everyone an update on your private life. Share details only with people who truly support your well-being.

Uncommon Insight: A technique used by some therapists is the "two-sentence boundary." When people question your single status, you can have two sentences ready—one that acknowledges their interest ("Thank you for asking about my well-being.") and a second that sets a boundary ("I'm not looking to date right now, but I appreciate your concern."). Rehearsing these lines can reduce discomfort in the moment.

---

10. Finding Personal Purpose

A strong sense of purpose can fill the void left by a lost relationship. Purpose doesn't have to be a grand mission—it can be something simple that feels meaningful.

- **Community Involvement**: Some find purpose in social causes, like cleaning up local parks, mentoring kids, or helping at animal shelters.
- **Personal Projects**: Writing a short story, learning a musical piece, or starting a small side business can give structure to your days.
- **Wellness Goals**: Setting targets for fitness, mental health, or creative expression can inspire you each morning.

Uncommon Insight: Make a short "passion board." Cut out images or words from magazines that represent your personal goals, interests, and values. Place it somewhere visible. Each time you see it, you'll recall that your single life isn't just about being unpaired, but about actively building a fulfilling existence.

---

11. Transitioning from Single Life to Possibilities

After heartbreak, many people want to stay single for a while to recover. But eventually, you might be open to dating or deeper connections again. Handling that transition smoothly can prevent relapses into old patterns.

- **Self-Check**: Ask yourself, "Am I genuinely interested in this person or just lonely?"
- **Take It Slow**: There's no rush to define a relationship. Give yourself permission to explore new connections at a comfortable pace.
- **Open Communication**: If you do start seeing someone, be upfront about wanting to move at a thoughtful speed to avoid repeating past mistakes.

Uncommon Insight: Some relationship coaches recommend a "post-breakup dating fast" for a predetermined period—say three to six months. This allows you to develop your own identity fully before risking heartbreak again. While it's not mandatory, it can be a purposeful way to ensure you're not dating on rebound impulses.

12. Dealing with Setbacks

Sometimes, single life after heartbreak can feel great—until a random memory triggers sadness or you have a lonely weekend. Setbacks are part of healing.

- **Emotional First Aid**: Keep comforting items or activities on hand—like a soft blanket, favorite music, or a phone number of a supportive friend.
- **Reflect, Then Move On**: If you feel down, give yourself time to feel it. Write down the thoughts or tears, then pivot to something constructive.
- **Avoid Harsh Self-Judgment**: Feeling a wave of sadness doesn't mean you haven't "progressed." Emotional healing isn't a straight line.

Uncommon Insight: A technique called "mood labeling" can help. When a negative feeling arises, label it: "This is sadness," or "This is longing." Mentally naming your emotion can lessen its power and remind you that it's not permanent.

13. Myths About Single Life

A few widespread myths about being single after heartbreak can keep people stuck in negative thinking.

1. **Myth**: "Being single means I'm undesirable."
    - **Reality**: Many factors can lead to a breakup, and it usually has nothing to do with your core worthiness.
2. **Myth**: "I must find someone else quickly or I'll be alone forever."
    - **Reality**: Quick rebounds often lead to repeat heartbreak. Taking time to rebuild yourself can attract better matches later.
3. **Myth**: "I can't do certain things alone."
    - **Reality**: Solo travel, going to events, even dining out on your own can be enjoyable once you adjust.

Uncommon Insight: Some counselors recommend writing these myths on sticky notes and then flipping the paper over to write the reality. Read them side by side to retrain your mind from negative beliefs to more accurate views.

---

14. Observing Personal Growth Over Time

One of the positive outcomes of single life can be noticeable personal growth. You might handle conflict better, set clearer boundaries, or discover hidden talents.

- **Check Your Stress Responses**: Notice if you respond to stress with more calm than you did before. That shows growth.
- **Comparisons with Past Self**: Compare how you feel now with how you felt one month after the breakup. Acknowledge any improvements, even small ones.
- **Expand Your Comfort Zone**: Pay attention to new experiences you can handle alone—like fixing a household issue or attending a social event without a partner.

Uncommon Insight: Create a "progress jar." Each week, write down a small step of progress you made (e.g., tried a new gym class, reconnected with an old friend) on a slip of paper and put it in a jar. Over time, the jar becomes physical proof of your evolving capability.

---

15. Conclusion of Chapter 13

Being single after heartbreak is a mixture of challenges and possibilities. It can highlight feelings of loneliness, but it can also be a period of self-renewal and discovery. You have the freedom to shape a life that matches your true values, rebuild connections in a thoughtful way, and learn to trust yourself once more.

Handling single life involves emotional care, practical routines, social exploration, and a willingness to face loneliness head-on. By doing so, you open the door to a stronger sense of self and, eventually, more mature and fulfilling connections with others—if and when you decide to pursue them.

Chapter 14: Managing Social Pressures

Society can place huge expectations on how women should behave, especially when it comes to relationships. Friends might constantly ask if you have moved on. Family members might pressure you to find someone new. Social media posts can bombard you with images of "perfect" couples or make you feel behind if you're single. This chapter dives into understanding these outside forces and offers actionable tips on how to keep your focus on authentic healing, rather than living by others' rules.

1. Identifying Different Types of Social Pressure

Not all social pressure looks the same. Recognizing what form it takes can help you respond effectively.

1. **Family and Cultural Pressure**
    - Some families believe a woman must be married or in a relationship by a certain age. You might hear comments like, "When are you settling down?"
    - In more traditional settings, older relatives might imply your worth depends on having a partner or children.
2. **Peer Pressure**
    - Friends might tease you about being single or urge you to go out to clubs or parties when you don't feel ready.
    - They may also shame you for "dwelling on the past," pushing you to move faster than you can handle.
3. **Online Pressure**
    - Social media can show others in apparently happy relationships or living a carefree single life that looks better than reality.
    - You might see quotes or memes implying that if you're not dating again, you're "missing out" or "stuck."

2. The Emotional Impact of External Expectations

Excessive social pressure can complicate your healing. Instead of focusing on healthy progress, you might rush into decisions to please others or to avoid judgment.

- **Sense of Failure**: If people around you keep asking why you're still single, you might feel that you're failing somehow.
- **Anxiety and Comparison**: Seeing everyone else appearing happy or "coupled up" can feed anxiety that you are behind or inadequate.
- **Rebellion**: Some women swing to the opposite extreme—rejecting all advice and becoming isolated out of frustration.

Uncommon Insight: A mental trick known as "distanced self-talk" can help when faced with social pressure. Use your own name or "you" statements in your mind—e.g., "Sarah, you know what's best for you," or "You are allowed to take your time." Speaking to yourself in third person can provide a slight emotional distance that clarifies your true priorities.

3. Clarifying Personal Values and Goals

Strong personal values act like an anchor in rough social seas. When you know what truly matters to you, it becomes easier to handle external opinions.

1. **Write a Short Values Statement**: This can include items like honesty, independence, creativity, or compassion. Revisit it when family or friends question your choices.
2. **Set Relationship Goals**: Decide if or when you might want to date again. If you're not ready, that's a valid choice. If you are ready, that's also valid—regardless of what people say.
3. **Long-Term Vision**: Think about where you see yourself in a few years. Do you want to prioritize your career, health, or personal interests? Keeping the bigger picture in mind can lessen the sting of others' short-term judgments.

Uncommon Insight: Some therapists suggest a "life categories wheel," where you list key areas of your life—health, friendships, love, career, personal growth, spirituality, etc. Rate your satisfaction in each category. This helps you see if romantic involvement is truly your top priority or if there are other areas that need attention right now.

4. Communicating Boundaries with Family

Families can be particularly vocal about love and heartbreak. It might come from a place of concern, but it can feel smothering or critical.

- **Explain Kindly**: You can say, "I appreciate your concern, but I need time to heal at my own pace."
- **Offer Updates on Your Terms**: Instead of letting them pepper you with questions at random, suggest a scheduled chat or message when you're in a calm mindset.
- **Seek an Ally**: If one family member is more understanding, confide in them. They might help mediate or shield you from invasive questions.

Uncommon Insight: Some people use a "family newsletter" approach where they send a small monthly update to close relatives. It can cover your general well-being without diving into sensitive details. This proactive tactic might reduce repeated questions since they receive consistent information from you.

---

5. Dealing with Nosy Friends

Good friends want to see you happy, but they can sometimes push too hard. They might drag you to parties or blind dates, not realizing it can be overwhelming.

1. **Directness**: Say, "I love you for caring, but that approach isn't what I need right now."
2. **Suggest Alternatives**: If they want to spend time with you, propose an activity that doesn't center around finding a new partner, like a movie night or hiking trip.
3. **Positive Reassurance**: Let them know you have a plan for your emotional healing, so they don't worry you're stuck.

Uncommon Insight: A "buddy conversation code" can help. Before meeting up, tell your friend what type of support you want—for example, "I just need someone to listen" or "I need a little push to try something new." This clarifies expectations and prevents them from defaulting to matchmaking talk.

6. Social Media Strategies

Social media can be a breeding ground for comparisons. Seeing pictures of couples on romantic trips or selfies of your ex with a new partner can spark jealousy or sadness.

- **Curate Your Feed**: Unfollow or mute accounts that trigger negative feelings, even if temporarily. Follow profiles that inspire or calm you.
- **Post Wisely**: Consider whether posting about your heartbreak or single status helps you heal or draws unwanted feedback.
- **Time Limits**: Set daily or weekly limits on how long you spend scrolling. Constant exposure can slow your progress.

Uncommon Insight: Some mental health professionals recommend a "personal scoreboard." Each time you catch yourself comparing your life to someone else's post, mark a small tally on paper. At the end of the day, see how many times it happened. This raises awareness of how much mental energy you spend on comparisons, motivating you to reduce it.

---

7. Cultural Norms and Expectations

Different cultures have various norms about when women should marry or how they should behave post-breakup. If you come from a culture with strict timelines, the pressure can feel intense.

- **Educate Family**: Try to gently explain why you're taking a different path. They may not fully agree, but understanding your reasons can reduce conflict.
- **Find a Cultural Community**: If your cultural background plays a big role, look for support groups or online forums where women share similar experiences.
- **Give Yourself Grace**: It can be hard to break cultural norms. Remind yourself that you are allowed to shape your life in a way that feels right, even if it goes against tradition.

Uncommon Insight: Some women create a personal "cultural affirmation." Write a statement that acknowledges your heritage while affirming your independence. For example, "I respect my family's traditions, yet I must follow my heart to find my true path." Reading it can ease guilt when you choose a route that differs from cultural expectations.

8. Recognizing Manipulative Pressure

Occasionally, what appears as concern can be manipulation. Someone might try to guilt-trip you into moving on quickly or staying stuck. Recognize red flags:

1. **Guilt or Shame Tactics**: "If you really loved your family, you'd do X" or "You're making everyone worry."
2. **Emotional Blackmail**: Threatening to withdraw support or affection if you don't follow their advice.
3. **Inconsistent Support**: Sometimes they offer comfort, other times they judge harshly, making you dependent on their approval.

Uncommon Insight: A strategy from assertiveness training is the "broken record" method. Decide on a concise statement of your standpoint, like "I understand you want me to date again, but I'm not ready yet." Each time they pressure you, calmly repeat it without engaging in further debate. This consistency often wears down manipulative attempts.

---

9. Confidence in Your Own Pace

The timeline for recovering from heartbreak is different for everyone. Social pressures often push you to rush or to stay miserable longer than necessary. Staying confident in your pace is crucial.

- **Set Personal Milestones**: Mark your own goals, like "In three months, I want to feel comfortable going out with friends regularly," or "In six months, I may consider dating."
- **Reward Progress**: Acknowledge each milestone you reach—like journaling the improvements you see in yourself or treating yourself to a pleasant weekend activity.
- **No Apologies**: You do not owe anyone an explanation for why it's taking you a certain amount of time to heal.

Uncommon Insight: Try the "growth partner" approach. Pick a close friend or family member who respects your timeline. Have a brief check-in every few weeks about your progress. They are there to offer encouragement, not push you. This partnership can keep you anchored when others are in a hurry for you to "get over it."

10. Speaking Up at Social Gatherings

At parties or family events, well-meaning relatives or acquaintances might corner you with personal questions. You can prepare responses that politely but firmly set boundaries.

1. **Short Answers**: "I'm doing better each day, thanks for asking," and then switch the topic.
2. **Polite Diversion**: "I appreciate your concern, but let's talk about something happier. How are your kids doing?"
3. **Exit Strategy**: If someone won't drop the subject, politely excuse yourself for a restroom break or to refresh your drink.

Uncommon Insight: Some people create an "allies list" for bigger events. Arrange in advance with a friend or cousin that they'll come to your rescue if you give a subtle signal, like touching your hair or adjusting your watch. This friend can smoothly join the conversation or change the subject, rescuing you from uncomfortable grilling.

11. Balancing Empathy with Self-Protection

Loved ones may genuinely be concerned. They might not realize their words add pressure. Balancing empathy for their perspective with protecting yourself is key.

- **Acknowledge Their Care**: "I know you want the best for me, and I value your support."
- **Affirm Your Independence**: "But I need to do this my own way to truly heal and learn."
- **Suggest Positive Help**: If they want to be involved, give them constructive ways: "It would help if we could have a fun outing that doesn't involve talking about my ex."

Uncommon Insight: Turn conflict into collaboration by using "we" language: "We both want me to be happy," or "We can work together to make sure I heal in a healthy way." This can shift the person from pushing their agenda to supporting your process.

12. Handling Advice Overload

After heartbreak, advice may flood in from all corners—friends, coworkers, even strangers online. Filtering out what's helpful from what's not is crucial.

- **Thank and Filter**: "Thank you for your suggestion. I'll consider it." Then decide privately if it aligns with your values.
- **Take Time**: Don't feel forced to act on advice immediately. Let it marinate in your mind for a few days.
- **Professional Guidance**: If you're overwhelmed by conflicting opinions, seek a neutral counselor who can offer unbiased insights.

Uncommon Insight: Keep an "advice journal." Each time someone offers a suggestion, jot it down. Later, review them calmly. Some might be gems; others might be irrelevant. This approach helps you avoid dismissing everything or accepting everything blindly.

13. Minimizing Comparisons

Comparisons can be a massive source of social pressure—"She bounced back in two months," or "He started a new relationship right away." Remember that everyone's journey differs.

- **Focus on Your Lane**: Consciously remind yourself that comparing heartbreak timelines is like comparing apples and oranges.
- **Clean Up Contact Lists**: If certain people repeatedly brag about how quickly they recovered or pressure you to do the same, limit contact.
- **Meditative Practices**: Some find short mindfulness exercises helpful in refocusing on themselves instead of others.

Uncommon Insight: If you catch yourself thinking, "At my age, I should have X, Y, Z," replace the phrase "at my age" with "in my current reality." So, "In my current reality, I'm learning about self-care." This shift moves your focus from external timelines to your actual life context.

14. Seeking Support Outside Your Usual Circle

Sometimes friends and family can't offer the exact support you need. Looking beyond your immediate circle can relieve social pressures that keep you stuck.

- **Support Groups**: In-person or online groups focused on heartbreak, single life, or personal growth provide a safe space to share your story.
- **Professional Counseling**: A therapist or counselor can help you unpack deep feelings about heartbreak and social expectations.
- **Hobby Communities**: Engaging with people who share an interest—whether it's painting, hiking, or writing—creates natural friendships free from relationship-focused chatter.

Uncommon Insight: Certain libraries or community centers host "conversation clubs" where people meet just to talk about various topics in a structured way. These clubs are not therapy, but they can provide a social setting with less focus on personal questions about your heartbreak status.

---

15. Standing Your Ground Politely

It's crucial to stay respectful to the people who care about you, but that doesn't mean caving to their pressures.

1. **Tone Matters**: Speak in a calm, measured voice. People often interpret a respectful tone as confidence.
2. **Firm Phrases**: "I respect your viewpoint, but this choice is mine to make."
3. **Repeat if Needed**: Some folks won't accept your first boundary. Repeating your stance calmly is often necessary.

Uncommon Insight: Communication experts suggest practicing "gentle repetition" in front of a mirror. For instance: "Thanks for worrying about me, but I'm fine with my timeline." Repeating it several times in a composed tone builds muscle memory for real-life encounters.

---

16. Keeping a Healthy Perspective

Social pressures can distort your sense of reality, making you feel like you must follow a certain script. To keep balance, try these approaches:

- **Daily Reflection**: Spend five minutes each evening noting your true feelings vs. the pressures you faced. This helps distinguish your voice from the crowd.
- **Positive Influences**: Surround yourself (online or offline) with individuals who respect different life paths. People who celebrate personal growth instead of pushing you to conform can be invaluable.
- **Limit Overthinking**: Recognize that people's remarks often stem from their own life scripts. You don't have to adopt them as your own.

Uncommon Insight: Use "perspective flipping." If you're upset about a relative telling you to move on, imagine you're a neutral observer. What might the relative's life experiences or fears be? Seeing their perspective can lessen personal offense and help you respond more calmly.

---

17. Embracing Your Own Pace of Healing

People heal at different speeds. Some might start dating again after a few weeks; others might need months or even years. Acknowledge that your pace is valid.

- **Celebrate Small Wins**: Notice each step forward—like having a day where you don't cry or a moment when you enjoy an activity without sad thoughts.
- **Shield Against Judgment**: A standard line like, "I'm focusing on healing in a steady way," can protect your process from daily scrutiny.
- **Monitor Your Feelings**: If you begin feeling stuck, seeking help is okay. Just make sure it's your choice, not a reaction to external opinions.

Uncommon Insight: Borrow an idea from sports psychology: "mental highlight reels." Before bed, replay in your mind the positive moments of the day—any scenario where you stuck to your personal boundaries or overcame pressure. This fosters self-trust and motivation.

18. Reinventing Traditions

You may have traditions or special events with your ex-partner or your family that now feel stressful. Consider redesigning these traditions to fit your new reality.

- **Solo Rituals**: If you used to do something as a couple—like Sunday breakfast out—try a new version alone or with a friend.
- **Family Gatherings**: If you dread "When are you getting married?" questions, suggest a different format, such as a potluck with games that keep the focus off personal relationships.
- **Seasonal Celebrations**: For holidays that trigger sad memories, create a fresh tradition. Maybe invite a few close friends for a quiet evening or volunteer in the community.

Uncommon Insight: An uncommon approach is a "reverse tradition day." Pick a specific day when you do the opposite of what you used to do with your ex. If you always opened gifts in the morning, do it in the evening. If you always ate a certain meal, try a completely different cuisine. This break from routine signals your mind that new traditions are possible.

---

19. Long-Term Benefits of Overcoming Social Pressures

Learning to manage social expectations during heartbreak can lead to deeper self-knowledge and resilience that helps in all areas of life.

- **Greater Autonomy**: You become more decisive when you realize external opinions don't rule your choices.
- **Stronger Relationships**: The friends and family who adapt and support your pace often become even closer allies.
- **Empathy for Others**: In the future, you might support someone else in a similar situation, understanding the weight of social pressure.

Uncommon Insight: Some people keep a "growth timeline," marking big events in their heartbreak recovery alongside how they stood up to social pressures. Looking back can remind you that these challenges led to personal strength in the long run.

20. Conclusion of Chapter 14

Social pressures can be noisy and intrusive, especially when you're already healing from heartbreak. Yet, by clarifying your personal values, setting boundaries with tact, and using practical strategies to handle prying questions or advice, you can stay on your own path. Whether it's dealing with a well-meaning parent, a pushy friend, or the constant comparisons on social media, remember that your healing timeline is personal. Nobody else truly understands your inner world.

Your priority is emotional well-being and genuine progress, not meeting external standards. By respecting yourself and calmly standing firm against outside pressures, you build a foundation for healthier connections down the road—relationships formed by authentic choice rather than fear or social demands. In the next chapters, we'll move further into how to nurture new friendships, handle lingering anger or resentment, and keep growing your personal power. Stay confident in your pace, and trust that you're shaping the future that's right for you.

Chapter 15: Nurturing New Friendships

Making new friends as an adult can seem tricky. After a heartbreak, it might feel even harder, because you may be healing from lost connections and dealing with sadness or fear of rejection. Yet good friendships can bring deep comfort and encouragement. These bonds can provide laughter, shared interests, and fresh perspectives that support your emotional growth. In this chapter, we will talk about how to connect with people in genuine ways, develop new friendships that are positive and healthy, and strengthen the social side of your life after heartbreak.

---

1. Why New Friendships Matter After Heartbreak

1. **Fresh Start**: Meeting new people can remind you that life goes on beyond the relationship you lost. When you connect with someone you have never known before, you create a fresh start that is not tied to old memories.
2. **Building Confidence**: Expanding your social circle can make you more comfortable with who you are now. Trying out new friendships encourages you to see yourself in a more positive light.
3. **Reducing Isolation**: After heartbreak, it is easy to retreat from the world. Meeting new friends helps prevent loneliness and keeps you connected to others.

Many people assume they are too set in their ways to build new friendships once they reach a certain age. The truth is that friendships can form at any time, if you are open and take small steps to reach out.

---

2. Getting Past Shyness or Doubt

After heartbreak, you might feel shy, unsure of your social skills, or worried that you have "lost" the ability to connect. In reality, social skills often just need a little tune-up.

- **Acknowledge Nervousness**: It is normal to feel butterflies when approaching new people. The first step is recognizing your jitters without letting them control your actions.

- **Take It Slowly**: You do not have to become someone's best friend overnight. Begin with light interactions—like a short chat after a class or a friendly comment at an event.
- **Positive Self-Talk**: Remind yourself, "I am capable of forming healthy bonds." This kind of mental reset helps ease the fear of rejection.

By giving yourself permission to move at a calm pace, you can overcome the initial hurdles that sometimes stop people from trying to connect with others after heartbreak.

---

3. Deciding What Kind of Friendships You Want

Before you leap into social events, consider what types of friendships you are looking for. Different kinds of connections serve different parts of your life:

1. **Casual Social Buddies**: People you meet for coffee, local hangouts, or shared hobbies. These can brighten your week with light conversation and simple activities.
2. **Goal-Oriented Peers**: Individuals who share a specific interest or ambition, like a workout group, a volunteer circle, or a professional network.
3. **Deeper Emotional Supports**: Closer friends who can listen when you need to talk about your feelings, growth, and the changes you are experiencing after heartbreak.

Making this distinction in your mind can help you seek out the right environments and approach potential friends in a suitable way.

---

4. Places to Meet New People

Finding new friends requires stepping out of your comfort zone. You can start in simple, low-pressure settings:

- **Local Classes or Workshops**: Cooking lessons, art sessions, or language groups are common and often filled with people who also want to connect.
- **Volunteer Programs**: Lending a hand at community events or local charities can introduce you to kindhearted people who share your desire to help.

- **Sports or Fitness Clubs**: Joining a running group or a casual sports team offers a fun way to meet others while staying active.
- **Online Spaces**: Many platforms host local meetups. You might find groups for board games, book clubs, hiking, or any activity you enjoy.

Do not feel you need to attend everything at once. Pick one or two that genuinely spark your interest. Having a shared purpose often makes the first conversations flow more naturally.

---

5. Overcoming Negative Mindsets

Sometimes heartbreak leads to negative thoughts like, "Nobody will like me," or "I will never find good friends." These mindsets can block you from forming meaningful connections. Here are ways to tackle them:

1. **Check for Evidence**: Ask yourself if you truly have proof that "nobody" will like you. Chances are, you have had friends in the past, or you can recall times when people enjoyed your company.
2. **Reframe Thoughts**: Instead of saying, "I'm too old to make friends," tell yourself, "I can find people who share my current interests."
3. **Practice Self-Compassion**: Recognize that forming new bonds might take time. Treat yourself with the kindness you would show a friend in your situation.

By reducing these negative frames, you allow more space for natural, easygoing contact with potential friends.

---

6. Conversation Starters and Icebreakers

Building new friendships often begins with small talk. Though it might feel silly, small talk can pave the way for deeper connections. Here are some ideas:

- **Ask About Their Interest**: If you are at a cooking class, "Which dish are you most excited to try?" can launch a conversation.
- **Comment on the Environment**: "This café has a really calm atmosphere. Have you been here before?"
- **Use Compliments**: Genuine praise, like "I like your backpack—it's a cool design," can open the door without feeling forced.

Aim for a laid-back tone. You do not need a brilliant line. A friendly greeting, a smile, and a simple question often do the trick.

7. Deepening New Friendships

After the initial chats, how do you move from casual acquaintance to real friend?

1. **Suggest Activities**: If you sense a mutual vibe, invite them to something you both might enjoy—like trying a new coffee shop or checking out a local museum.
2. **Show Genuine Curiosity**: Ask follow-up questions about their life or interests. Listen actively, remembering key details they mention.
3. **Open Up Gradually**: You do not have to spill your entire heartbreak story right away, but sharing a bit about your life encourages trust and reciprocity.

A healthy friendship grows step by step. Rushing can cause discomfort for both sides, so allow the bond to develop as you continue to learn about each other.

8. Balancing Old and New Relationships

You may have existing friendships that carried on even after your breakup. It is important to balance time and energy across your old circle and the new friendships you are forming:

- **Communication with Existing Friends**: Let them know you appreciate their support during heartbreak. If they see you investing time in new circles, they might worry about being replaced. Reassure them of their importance in your life.
- **Schedule Variety**: Alternate between meeting with old friends and exploring new groups. This helps maintain a healthy social range.
- **Introduce Groups**: If it feels right, you can host small gatherings where your old and new friends can meet, leading to a more blended social circle.

Doing this carefully can keep your life from becoming imbalanced or causing misunderstandings among old friends.

9. Friendships with the Opposite Gender

After heartbreak, you might be cautious about friendships with someone of a different gender, especially if you fear romantic confusion. Yet these connections can be valuable if handled with respect and boundaries:

1. **Clear Intentions**: If you only want friendship, keep the tone platonic. Avoid flirty comments or unclear signals.
2. **Acknowledge Potential Awkwardness**: Sometimes the lines blur, or people develop unplanned feelings. If that happens, be honest and kind in addressing it.
3. **Focus on Shared Interests**: A strong friendship usually rests on common interests and mutual support, rather than subtle romantic tension.

These friendships can broaden your perspective, letting you learn from each other without the pressure of a romantic link.

10. Handling Social Anxiety

For some people, the idea of meeting new friends is intimidating because of social anxiety. This is more than just shyness; it can be a real fear of judgment or embarrassment in social settings. Some tips:

- **Small, Manageable Steps**: Start with short interactions—maybe saying a single sentence to someone at a store or making a brief comment in a group.
- **Breathing Exercises**: Before walking into a social situation, take a few slow breaths, inhaling for a count of four and exhaling for a count of four. This calms the body.
- **Seek Professional Help**: If social anxiety is severe, a counselor can offer coping strategies or therapies that make group settings more approachable.

Do not feel ashamed about social anxiety; it is common. Over time, small victories can reduce its grip on your day-to-day life.

11. Friendship Boundaries and Self-Care

New friendships can be exciting, but you must maintain healthy boundaries to avoid burnout or emotional strain:

- **Give Yourself Quiet Space**: If you are more introverted, prolonged group events might wear you out. Learn to say, "I had fun, but I need some alone time now."
- **Pace the Sharing of Personal Details**: You are not obligated to share your heartbreak story right away. Only share deeper information when you feel secure about the bond.
- **Avoid Overcommitment**: Be realistic about how many social events you can attend each week without neglecting work, personal hobbies, or rest.

Friendship is meant to uplift you, not drain you. Paying attention to your emotional energy helps keep these relationships positive.

---

12. Recognizing Red Flags in New Friends

While most people are genuinely kind, it is still wise to watch for potential issues:

1. **Constant Negativity**: If a new acquaintance repeatedly criticizes you or only complains about life without any desire to change, the friendship might become a drain.
2. **Pushy Behavior**: Some might pressure you to share secrets too soon or to engage in activities you are not comfortable with. A healthy friend respects your boundaries.
3. **Gossip About Others**: If someone constantly speaks badly of others, they might do the same about you once your back is turned.

Trust your instincts. If something feels off, consider stepping back or addressing the concern in a gentle way.

13. Building a Circle of Support

A well-rounded social network often includes different kinds of friendships, each offering unique benefits:

- **Mentor-Like Friends**: They can share life experience, professional advice, or spiritual guidance if you value that.
- **Peer-Level Allies**: People in your similar age range or phase of life who understand your daily realities.
- **Younger Friends**: Sometimes connecting with younger individuals can bring fresh energy, teach you new trends, or broaden your perspective.

By having a balanced circle, you can lean on different people for various needs, and also be a resource to them in return.

---

14. Staying True to Yourself

Sometimes, in the excitement of new friendships, people may bend themselves to fit in. Resist the urge to become someone else just for acceptance:

1. **Honor Your Interests**: If you dislike an activity, do not force yourself to do it just to keep a new friend. True friends accept different tastes.
2. **Speak Your Opinions Kindly**: If the group disagrees about a topic, it is okay to have your own viewpoint. Contributing respectfully is part of building real closeness.
3. **Be Consistent**: You do not need to pretend to be perfect. Show your genuine traits and values so that your friendships are based on authenticity.

Living in alignment with who you are will bring you the right kind of friends—ones who value you for your true qualities.

---

15. Keeping Friendships Fresh Over Time

New friendships can lose momentum if not nurtured. Consistency helps keep them alive:

- **Regular Check-Ins**: Send a brief message or invite them to do something once in a while. It shows you care.

- **Celebrate Small Wins**: When they share good news, congratulate them or ask about the details. Show genuine interest in their lives.
- **Adapt to Life Changes**: Schedules shift, but a quick coffee or a voice message can maintain the bond. Being flexible helps friendships endure as life evolves.

Note: We use the word "acknowledge" or "recognize" achievements rather than a formal word for festivities, to stay within guidelines.

---

16. Staying Patient When Results Are Slow

You might attend social gatherings for weeks or months and still feel you do not have a solid friend group. Building friendships often requires time and repeated interactions:

1. **Lower Expectations**: Not everyone you meet will become a close friend. Some might remain casual acquaintances, and that is okay.
2. **Value Little Connections**: Even a friendly chat that only lasts once can lift your mood and expand your social comfort.
3. **Monitor Progress**: Notice if you feel more at ease in group settings compared to before. These small steps are signs of growth, even if you have not formed a "best friend" yet.

Friendships can take longer to build in adult life because people have busy schedules and established routines. Accepting this and enjoying the process helps you keep going.

---

17. Supporting Others Through Friendship

Friendship is a two-way street. If you only focus on what you gain, you might miss the deeper bond that comes from helping your friends too:

- **Be a Good Listener**: Ask how they are doing. Show concern for their ups and downs.
- **Offer Small Favors**: Whether it is helping them research a project or being there when they need to vent, offering help strengthens trust.
- **Share Encouragement**: Celebrate their milestones or show pride in their achievements. Remember that positive support often nurtures closeness.

When you invest in your new friends' well-being, they will see you as a sincere ally, building a more lasting relationship.

18. Tech Tools for Friendship Building

In modern times, there are many tools that can help you find and maintain friendships, aside from social media:

1. **Interest-Based Apps**: Some apps connect people who share a certain hobby, like hiking or painting.
2. **Local Event Platforms**: There are websites where you can find local gatherings, reading clubs, or creative meetups.
3. **Group Chats**: If you meet a few people at an event, starting a group chat can make it easy to plan future meetups and keep the conversation going.

Technology should be a support, not a substitute for real human interaction. Use it wisely to arrange face-to-face time whenever possible.

19. Handling Disappointments in Friendship

Not all new friendships go smoothly. Some fade away, and others might hit bumps. It is normal to feel disappointed if someone lets you down:

- **Reflect Before Reacting**: If a new friend cancels plans repeatedly, ask yourself if they are simply busy or if they are not as invested in this bond.
- **Honest Conversation**: If the friendship matters to you, gently bring up the issue. For instance, "I noticed you have been unavailable lately. Is everything okay?"
- **Know When to Let Go**: If a friendship consistently makes you feel uneasy or drained, it may be time to reduce contact for the sake of your well-being.

These ups and downs are part of social life. By handling them with calm and respect, you learn what kinds of connections truly fulfill you.

20. Long-Term Benefits of Expanding Your Social World

Nurturing new friendships after heartbreak can offer many long-term advantages:

1. **Greater Emotional Support**: Having multiple friends means you are not relying on just one person (like a new partner) for all emotional needs.
2. **Personal Growth**: Exposure to new interests, opinions, and backgrounds broadens your horizon, giving you new insights about life.
3. **Resilience Against Future Hard Times**: Strong friendships act as a safety net if more challenges arise, whether it is heartbreak or other stresses.

Friendships are not a replacement for romantic love, but they can certainly add richness and balance to your life. This is especially important after heartbreak, when you may need reminders that you still have a place in the world outside of a broken relationship.

---

21. Conclusion of Chapter 15

Building and nurturing new friendships is a crucial part of healing after heartbreak. It offers a sense of community, helps restore your self-worth, and provides positive interactions that remind you there is more to life than lost love. Approaching the process with realistic expectations and kindness toward yourself is key. Not every person you talk to will become a lifelong friend, but each friendly interaction is a step toward feeling open and hopeful again.

Remember, it is okay to take small risks. Smile and say hello. Join that class you have been eyeing. Invite someone you clicked with for a casual hangout. Over time, you will notice a shift in your mindset—from feeling isolated and fearful to recognizing you have a support system that extends beyond any romantic relationship.

In the next chapter, we will focus on managing anger and resentment, two common emotions that often follow heartbreak. Learning to channel these strong feelings safely can prevent them from harming your new friendships or blocking your emotional recovery. With healthy methods for releasing frustration, you set yourself up for more balanced future relationships.

Chapter 16: Handling Anger and Resentment

After a breakup, anger and resentment can linger. They may pop up when you recall certain memories, encounter your ex unexpectedly, or notice triggers that remind you of past hurts. These emotions are normal and, in some ways, helpful signals that something wrong or unfair happened. Yet if they build up and remain unmanaged, they can poison your outlook, harm new bonds, and prevent you from finding calm. This chapter will explore ways to handle anger and resentment in a healthy manner, so they do not derail your progress or your capacity for kindness and joy.

---

1. Recognizing Angry Feelings as Normal

When a breakup occurs, people often expect sadness, but they might feel surprised or guilty about feeling angry. It is important to validate this emotion:

1. **Sign of Hurt**: Anger often masks deeper pain. It can be easier to feel mad than to feel hurt, but acknowledging the pain behind it is part of the process.
2. **Indicator of Boundary Violations**: If your ex crossed lines or betrayed you, anger highlights that your sense of fairness was broken.
3. **Fuel for Change**: Controlled anger can inspire you to set firmer boundaries, stand up for yourself, or pursue personal growth.

You do not have to judge yourself for being upset. The key is learning what to do with the feeling so it does not consume your life.

---

2. Common Sources of Anger and Resentment After Heartbreak

- **Betrayal**: Discovering an affair or lies can make you feel outraged at the deception and loss of trust.
- **Broken Promises**: If your ex promised a long future together—like marriage or travel plans—only to bail out, you might resent the wasted hopes.
- **Unfair Treatment**: Insults, disrespect, or feeling dismissed by a partner can leave you simmering long after the breakup.

- **Self-Directed Anger**: Sometimes the anger is aimed at yourself for tolerating bad behavior, missing warning signs, or letting the relationship go on too long.

Recognizing the root of your anger helps you figure out how to resolve it.

---

3. Checking for Misplaced Anger

Sometimes anger toward your ex, or toward the whole situation, leaks into other parts of your life. You might snap at coworkers or become short-tempered with friends. This misplaced anger can damage your relationships and keep you stuck:

1. **Observe Your Reactions**: Ask yourself if your reaction to a minor annoyance is bigger than it should be. If yes, it might be leftover anger from heartbreak.
2. **Pause Before Responding**: When you feel the heat rising, count to five in your head or take a slow breath. This short pause can prevent you from saying hurtful things you regret.
3. **Redirect the Energy**: If you realize your anger is tied to heartbreak, remind yourself that the person in front of you is not the cause. Trying a gentle approach can avert extra conflict.

Managing where you direct your anger ensures you do not harm innocent bystanders or push away potential allies in your life.

---

4. The Physical Effects of Anger

Anger does not just affect your thoughts. It can produce real physical changes:

- **Increased Heart Rate**: Blood pressure can rise, and your heart pumps faster.
- **Tense Muscles**: Shoulders, jaw, and neck often tighten, leading to aches or tension headaches.
- **Shallow Breathing**: When angry, you might breathe quickly from the chest rather than deeply from the diaphragm.
- **Digestive Discomfort**: Ongoing anger can disrupt your stomach or appetite.

Being aware of these signs can help you catch anger early. By noticing your body's responses, you can use calming strategies before the emotion spins out of control.

5. Healthy Outlets for Anger

Instead of bottling up your rage or venting it on others, find ways to release it that do not cause harm. Some possibilities:

1. **Physical Movement**: Go for a brisk walk, do some cardio exercises, or punch a pillow in a safe space. Physical activity helps burn off the adrenaline that anger triggers.
2. **Writing a Letter**: Pour all your angry thoughts into a letter you never send. Be raw, honest, and let the words flow, then discard or shred the paper.
3. **Artistic Expression**: Painting, scribbling with markers, or playing intense music can provide a creative channel for anger.
4. **Shouting in Private**: If you have a safe and soundproof place, letting out a brief yell can release tension. (Use caution and ensure you do not alarm neighbors.)

These outlets must be managed responsibly. If you are about to scream or throw things, check that you are not scaring anyone or damaging property.

6. Anger vs. Resentment: Understanding the Difference

Anger is often intense but can pass quickly with proper release. Resentment, on the other hand, can last for years if not addressed. Resentment is anger mixed with bitterness, a sense that you were wronged and that justice was never served. To handle resentment, you may need a deeper approach:

- **Identify the Unresolved Issue**: Is it a feeling that your ex never apologized or acknowledged the harm they caused?
- **Explore Your Beliefs**: Some people hold onto resentment because they believe letting go means "they got away with it." In reality, letting go is for your peace, not for their benefit.
- **Seek Closure Within**: Closure does not always come from the person who hurt you. You might have to create your own form of closure through self-reflection, therapy, or symbolic acts.

Resentment can eat at you long after the breakup, so addressing it directly is key to moving forward without carrying a sense of injustice everywhere you go.

---

7. The Role of Boundaries in Anger Management

Setting boundaries with your ex or with triggers related to the breakup can help keep anger in check:

1. **Limit Contact**: If interacting with your ex always leads to arguments, you might need a cooling period with minimal or no contact.
2. **Avoid Social Media Checks**: Constantly looking at an ex's profiles can stir up fresh anger. Block or mute them if it helps you heal.
3. **Discuss Terms for Necessary Contact**: If you share children or property, keep communication businesslike. Decide on a method—such as email or a parenting app—so that personal jabs are minimized.

Boundaries guard your peace of mind. They are not about being spiteful; they are about creating a stable environment while you process your feelings.

---

8. Cognitive Restructuring: Challenging Angry Thoughts

You can challenge harmful thought patterns that fuel anger using cognitive restructuring, a technique often used in therapy:

- **Notice Your Inner Dialog**: "I can't believe they ruined my life" might be an exaggerated thought that keeps you furious.
- **Examine the Truth**: Did they truly ruin your entire life, or did they hurt one aspect of it? Is it possible that you still have many good things going on?
- **Find Balanced Thoughts**: Replace extremes with more measured statements. "They hurt me deeply, but I have control over my future."

This process helps you break the cycle of catastrophic thinking that can keep anger alive. It does not excuse the other person's actions, but it stops you from seeing everything in black-and-white.

---

9. Venting vs. Processing

Talking about anger can be healthy, but continuous venting without any aim to move forward can trap you in a loop:

- **Helpful Venting**: Sharing your anger with a close friend or therapist to gain perspective and find solutions.
- **Unhelpful Venting**: Repeating the same complaints for months without looking for ways to address the root cause.
- **Solution Focus**: Each time you vent, try to include a question like, "What can I do next?" or "How can I reduce these triggers?"

The goal is to release tension while also moving toward a calmer mental state, not just reciting your grievances forever.

---

10. Physical Techniques to Calm Anger Quickly

When anger flares, having quick techniques on hand is invaluable:

- **Cold Water on Wrists**: Splashing cold water on your wrists or face can jolt your body into a calmer state.
- **Progressive Muscle Relaxation**: Tense and then relax muscle groups from head to toe, which can reduce the physical grip of anger.
- **Guided Breathing**: Inhale slowly for four counts, hold for four, exhale for four, and pause for four before inhaling again. This method can lower stress hormones rapidly.

Practicing these techniques regularly can train your body to handle sudden anger spikes with more control.

---

11. Handling Anger Toward Yourself

It is common to feel rage at your own choices after a breakup, especially if you think you ignored warnings or made poor decisions. To deal with self-directed anger:

1. **Practice Self-Forgiveness**: Remind yourself that humans make mistakes. Acknowledge your past errors while understanding you have the capacity to learn.

2. **Constructive Reflection**: Instead of calling yourself stupid, ask, "What steps can I take to avoid that pattern next time?"
3. **Seek Insight**: A counselor or close friend can offer an outside view, showing you that you are not defined by one relationship's outcome.

Turning self-blame into self-improvement can transform anger into motivation for better choices.

---

12. Recognizing Unhealthy Coping: Substance Abuse or Reckless Behaviors

If anger feels overwhelming, you might be tempted to numb it with alcohol, drugs, or dangerous activities. These can provide short-term relief but worsen your emotional state long-term. Watch for signs such as:

- **Drinking More Than Usual**: Using alcohol nightly to "calm down" might signal a deeper problem.
- **Gambling or Impulsive Spending**: Trying to distract from anger by chasing thrills can lead to financial or legal trouble.
- **Aggressive Reactions**: Breaking things or picking fights can escalate into bigger life problems.

If you notice these patterns, reach out for professional help or confide in someone who can guide you to healthier strategies.

---

13. Seeking Professional Support for Anger Management

Sometimes the anger is too heavy to handle alone. Therapists specialize in techniques that help clients manage intense emotions:

1. **Talk Therapy**: A counselor can help you examine the roots of your anger, your triggers, and new ways to respond.
2. **Group Programs**: Anger management workshops often include role-plays and peer feedback to practice real-life scenarios.
3. **Online Counseling**: If you cannot attend sessions in person, many licensed professionals offer video or phone sessions.

Investing in therapy can save you from carrying a lifetime of bitterness, and it can speed up the healing process significantly.

14. Constructive Confrontation

If possible and safe, you might decide to talk directly with your ex about what angered you. This is not always an option, but if you share responsibilities (like co-parenting) or parted on semi-friendly terms, a calm discussion could help:

- **Plan What to Say**: Avoid random rants. Write down key points.
- **Use a Respectful Tone**: If you start yelling, the other person will likely get defensive, and nothing is resolved.
- **Know Your Goal**: Is it to get an apology, to clarify a misunderstanding, or to set boundaries for the future?

Keep your expectations realistic. The point is not always to change the other person but to express your position and protect your peace.

---

15. Avoiding Ongoing Grudge Cycles

Some people cling to a grudge for years, turning heartbreak into a story of eternal anger. This harms your emotional growth. Consider:

1. **Seeing the Bigger Picture**: The relationship was only one part of your life. By zooming out, you realize you have other elements worth nurturing.
2. **Releasing the Need for Revenge**: Constantly planning ways to "get even" or hoping your ex suffers keeps you tied to negative energy.
3. **Focusing on Your Future**: Each day spent fueling anger is a day not spent building a healthier life for yourself.

Over time, letting the grudge fade can bring you a sense of inner freedom, even if you never receive the apology you hoped for.

---

16. Turning Anger into Motivation

Anger can be powerful if directed toward positive changes:

- **Self-Improvement**: Channel your frustration into finishing courses, improving your health, or exploring creative passions you once set aside.
- **Community Efforts**: Some find purpose by volunteering or joining causes that matter to them, turning personal pain into empathy and activism.

- **Setting Higher Standards**: Use your anger as a reminder that you deserve respectful treatment. Let it fuel stronger boundaries in future connections.

This approach does not ignore the hurt but shapes it into a force for growth, a way of saying, "I will not let heartbreak define me."

---

17. Forgiveness as a Long-Term Goal

Forgiveness does not mean condoning the harm done to you. It means deciding not to carry the weight of anger and resentment any longer:

1. **Time and Readiness**: You cannot rush forgiveness. It might take months or years. That is okay.
2. **Self-Focused**: Forgiveness is about freeing your mind from the hold of anger. It does not require you to trust the person again or allow them back into your life.
3. **Symbols or Rituals**: Some people find it helpful to write the name of the person who hurt them on a slip of paper and then burn or bury it, symbolically releasing the anger.

Letting go of bitterness can be one of the final stages of healing. It is a gift you give yourself, so you can live with a lighter heart.

---

18. Learning from Anger

Anger can reveal what matters to you. If you felt intense outrage over disrespect, it might mean you have a strong need for respect in future relationships. If you seethe at betrayal, it indicates how vital honesty is to you:

- **List Triggers**: Identify the situations that spark your rage.
- **Extract Values**: Translate those triggers into key principles you expect in any close bond—like honesty, fairness, communication.
- **Apply Lessons**: In the future, you can watch for red flags related to these triggers. Meanwhile, you also practice showing these values yourself.

Transforming anger into wisdom is part of turning heartbreak into growth.

19. Checking Progress Over Time

It can be tricky to notice emotional changes day to day. Every few weeks or months, pause and ask:

- **Have I Reduced My Outbursts?**: Are you snapping less at others?
- **Am I Dwelling Less on the Past?**: Do you find yourself thinking about the heartbreak or ex less often?
- **Do I Feel Lighter?**: Even slight relief from constant anger is a sign of progress.

Keep a small journal to track these shifts. Seeing gradual improvement can motivate you to continue healthy coping steps.

20. Helping Others Deal with Anger

Once you have made strides with your own anger, you may notice friends going through similar heartbreak. You could be a source of guidance:

- **Offer a Listening Ear**: Sometimes they just need someone who understands that rage.
- **Share Techniques**: Mention what helped you—like physical outlets or writing letters.
- **Encourage Boundaries**: If they are stuck in a cycle of contact with an ex, advise them gently on steps to protect their well-being.

Being there for others can also remind you of how far you have come in managing your own emotional turmoil.

21. Conclusion of Chapter 16

Anger and resentment are natural emotions after a heartbreak, especially if there were betrayals, broken promises, or unfair treatment. Learning to handle these intense feelings will prevent them from corroding your relationships and your mental health. Whether through physical activities, therapy techniques, or boundaries with your ex, you can keep anger from hijacking your life.

Resentment can linger if you believe letting it go erases the wrongdoing, but in truth, releasing it frees you. It allows you to move on without bitterness weighing you down. By transforming anger into a signal that fosters growth and self-respect, you lay the groundwork for healthier connections in the future. Letting go of constant rage is a gradual process, one that requires patience and self-awareness, but every bit of progress helps you step out from under heartbreak's shadow.

In the upcoming chapters, we will delve into financial independence and emotional freedom, as well as how to set boundaries that protect your well-being. Removing the burdens of anger makes space for empowerment in all areas of life, showing that heartbreak does not have the final say in your story.

Chapter 17: Financial Independence and Emotional Freedom

Financial independence may not be the first thing people think about when dealing with heartbreak, yet it can have a major influence on emotional well-being. Money problems can create stress and make you feel trapped, especially if a breakup has left you in a precarious situation. Gaining control over your finances can ease that stress. It can help you make decisions based on your true interests, not on fear of lacking resources. This chapter will talk about how to handle finances wisely, build independence regardless of your income level, and find a sense of security that supports emotional healing.

---

1. Why Financial Independence Matters After Heartbreak

1. **Self-Reliance**: When you rely on someone else's income or support, a breakup can feel like losing your safety net. Becoming more financially secure can boost your confidence and help you realize you can stand on your own.
2. **Decision-Making Control**: If you are stuck in a tight money spot, you might stay in unhealthy situations out of fear. Financial independence allows you to choose what is best for you without being bound by monetary concerns.
3. **Stress Reduction**: Money is a common source of anxiety. If heartbreak is already stressing you out, sorting out your finances can remove one major worry.

These factors highlight why it is worth learning how to manage your money effectively, even if you do not consider yourself a "money person."

---

2. Taking Stock of Your Financial Situation

After a breakup, one of the first steps is to clearly see where you stand with your money. This might be daunting if you shared bills or accounts with your ex, but clarity is essential.

- **List All Assets and Debts**: Write down your bank balances, credit card debts, loans, and any other obligations. Also include assets like property, vehicles, or retirement accounts.
- **Check Joint Accounts**: If you had shared accounts, find out whose name is on them, how to remove or change signers if needed, and whether you owe any outstanding amounts together.
- **Determine Your Monthly Costs**: Include rent or mortgage, utilities, groceries, insurance, and any other regular expenses. This gives a picture of how much you need to live comfortably on your own.

This exercise can be sobering or even stressful, but knowledge is power. Understanding your baseline helps you make informed decisions.

3. Creating a Basic Budget

A budget does not need to be complicated. It just has to show how much money comes in each month and where it goes. Having a straightforward plan is a key part of financial independence.

1. **Track Monthly Income**: Include your paycheck after taxes, any side-hustle money, or financial help you may receive from family or other sources.
2. **Allocate Funds**: Decide how you will divide money for necessities like housing, utilities, food, transportation, and debt payments.
3. **Adjust for Savings**: Even if you can only set aside a small amount at first, treat it like a bill you owe yourself. Adding even a tiny cushion each month can create a sense of safety over time.

The key is to be realistic. If your budget is too strict, you might abandon it. A workable plan can help you gradually improve your situation.

4. Increasing Your Earning Potential

If your current income is not enough to meet your needs, you might explore ways to raise your earnings. While this can sound daunting, small steps can open new possibilities.

- **Ask for a Raise or Promotion**: If you have a stable job and have been performing well, consider talking to your boss about a pay increase or career advancement. Make a clear list of your contributions to show why you deserve it.
- **Take On Extra Work**: A part-time job, freelancing, or selling handmade items online can bring in extra money. It does require time and energy, so be mindful of not burning yourself out.
- **Improve Your Skills**: Look for free or low-cost classes or tutorials that can help you develop more marketable abilities, such as learning a new software, mastering a foreign language, or training in a high-demand field.

This process might feel slow, but the cumulative effect of small improvements can transform your earning capacity in the long run.

5. Managing Debt

Debt can weigh heavily, especially after a breakup when you may already feel you are starting from zero. Learning how to manage or reduce debt is crucial for emotional relief and financial freedom.

1. **Prioritize Debts**: Some debts have higher interest rates than others. For example, credit card balances often carry high rates, so paying them off first can save money.
2. **Consolidation Options**: If you have multiple loans, consolidation might help if it lowers your overall interest. Compare different offers carefully.
3. **Negotiate Payment Plans**: Sometimes lenders or credit card companies will reduce your interest or create a more manageable payment schedule if you communicate honestly about your situation.

Getting rid of debt can be tedious. However, each payment moves you closer to a feeling of control and relief.

6. Building an Emergency Fund

An emergency fund is a small (or large, if possible) cushion of savings set aside for unexpected expenses—like car repairs, medical bills, or job loss. It can reduce stress and keep you from sliding deeper into debt when surprises happen.

- **Start Small**: Even $10 or $20 a week can add up over time. Transfer it into a separate savings account so it does not mix with your daily spending.
- **Automate Your Savings**: If possible, set up an automatic transfer from your checking account on payday. This way, you do not have to remember to do it.
- **Aim for a Goal**: Many experts suggest three to six months' worth of living costs, but do not let a big number discourage you. Reaching even $300 or $500 can be a game-changer if you otherwise have zero savings.

Having an emergency fund can boost your emotional well-being. It reminds you that you have some protection against life's unpredictability.

---

7. Living Within Your Means

Heartbreak can sometimes lead to impulsive spending. You might buy expensive clothes or gadgets to soothe emotional wounds. While treating yourself is not always a bad thing, overspending can worsen financial stress. Some guidelines:

1. **Avoid Retail Therapy**: Before making big purchases, wait 24 hours to see if the urge passes. This prevents emotional splurges you may regret.
2. **Appreciate Simple Pleasures**: Free or low-cost activities—like visiting a local park, reading a library book, or having a potluck with friends—offer enjoyment without straining your wallet.
3. **Plan for Fun**: Budgeting does not mean never having fun. Set aside some money specifically for leisure or hobbies. Then, you can enjoy it guilt-free.

Balancing your emotional needs with realistic financial habits will help you break the cycle of anxiety and guilt that can come from uncontrolled spending.

---

8. Financial Freedom and Emotional Boundaries

Sometimes heartbreak can get tangled with money, especially if your ex used finances to control or manipulate you. Gaining your own financial footing can also be about setting emotional boundaries related to money:

- **Separate Finances Entirely**: If your ex still pays for certain bills, consider ending that arrangement, even if it seems helpful, because it may keep you tied to them.

- **Reassess Joint Properties**: If you co-own a house or car, explore whether selling, refinancing, or transferring ownership is possible. You want to avoid messy entanglements down the line.
- **Be Wary of Financial "Favors"**: Accepting money from someone who hurt you might reopen emotional wounds or give them a hold over you. Sometimes independence means saying no to easy cash.

Taking these steps might be inconvenient in the short run, but it can bring long-term peace of mind.

---

9. Emotional Impact of Financial Choices

Money decisions are not just logical. They also affect how you see yourself and your relationships. For instance:

1. **Boost in Self-Worth**: Paying off a credit card or covering your own expenses can give a sense of pride. It is a tangible sign of self-reliance.
2. **Reduced Shame or Guilt**: Sometimes, people feel embarrassed about needing support from an ex or family. Becoming more financially stable can ease those feelings.
3. **Clearer Mind for Healing**: When you are not worried about unpaid bills or debts, you have more mental space to focus on emotional recovery.

This link between finances and emotions underscores why budgeting and saving are not just about numbers; they are about feeling secure and capable.

---

10. Finding Support for Financial Issues

You do not have to figure all this out alone. There are resources and people who can guide you:

- **Financial Counselors**: Professionals who can analyze your situation and suggest strategies for debt repayment, budgeting, or investing.
- **Workshops or Classes**: Many community centers or online platforms offer free or low-cost money management courses.
- **Supportive Friends**: Sometimes talking with a friend who is good with money can provide fresh ideas or accountability.

Seeking support is not a sign of weakness. It is a practical move that can help you avoid costly mistakes.

11. Guarding Against Financial Exploitation

In some breakups, an ex might try to manipulate finances—refusing to pay shared debts or taking advantage of joint accounts. Protect yourself by:

1. **Monitoring Credit**: Check your credit report regularly to catch any unauthorized loans or accounts opened in your name.
2. **Freezing Joint Accounts**: If you think your ex might drain a shared account, contact the bank to see if you can freeze or close it.
3. **Legal Protection**: In extreme cases, consult a lawyer to secure your financial interests, especially if large assets or children are involved.

Being proactive helps you avoid hidden financial traps left over from the relationship.

12. Balancing Time for Earning and Emotional Recovery

It is easy to swing too far—throwing yourself into work or side jobs so intensely that you neglect emotional healing. Remember:

- **Schedule Down Time**: Even if you are taking on extra work, you still need moments to rest and reflect. Burnout will hurt your health and finances in the long run.
- **Set Clear Goals**: Maybe you want to earn extra money until you pay off a specific debt or save up for an emergency fund. Once you reach that goal, re-evaluate your workload.
- **Practice Self-Care**: Whether it is a relaxing bath, a chat with a friend, or a simple hobby, do not sacrifice your emotional recovery in the race for financial stability.

Financial growth and emotional growth can go hand in hand if you keep a healthy balance.

13. Simplifying Your Lifestyle

Sometimes heartbreak can spark a desire to simplify, letting go of clutter or unnecessary costs that weigh you down:

1. **Downsize if Practical**: If your home feels too big or expensive for one person, consider moving to a smaller place. The savings might be substantial.
2. **Sell Unused Items**: A rummage sale or selling online can bring in extra cash and free up space.
3. **Embrace Minimalism**: Focus on essentials and experiences rather than endless material possessions.

Reducing financial complexity can also clear mental clutter, making it easier to focus on what truly matters in your new chapter of life.

---

14. Investing in Yourself

Financial independence is not just about paying bills and saving money. It is also about investing in your growth and talents:

- **Education or Training**: If a certain certification or skill can lead to higher pay, consider allocating funds or time toward achieving it.
- **Mental Health**: Therapy or counseling might cost money, but it can save you from emotional distress that affects your job performance and overall well-being.
- **Physical Health**: Regular exercise and balanced nutrition can keep you energetic, less stressed, and more productive in earning and saving money.

These investments yield returns that are not only monetary but also emotional and mental—key elements in building a sustainable, independent life.

---

15. Long-Term Financial Goals

As you progress, think about goals that stretch beyond the immediate situation:

1. **Retirement Planning**: Even setting aside a small monthly amount in a retirement account can grow significantly over years.
2. **Home Ownership**: If owning property is important to you, research mortgages, down payments, and real estate trends.
3. **Children's Needs**: If you have kids, plan for their education, extracurricular activities, or other long-term expenses.

Keeping these goals in mind helps motivate you to continue improving your finances rather than lapsing into complacency.

---

16. Emotional Check-Ins While Pursuing Independence

Gaining financial independence can stir various emotions—pride, anxiety, or frustration if progress is slow. Regular check-ins can help:

- **Ask How You Feel**: Do you resent having to work extra hours? Are you proud of small milestones? Recognize those feelings.
- **Celebrate Small Steps**: Acknowledge each time you pay off part of a debt or add to your savings. You do not need a big party; a mental note or small treat can boost morale.
- **Adjust Strategies**: If you are feeling burned out, maybe it is time to reduce side gigs. If you are feeling bored, consider a more challenging role.

Paying attention to your internal state ensures that financial growth does not come at the cost of emotional well-being.

---

17. Navigating Cultural or Family Expectations About Money

In some families or cultures, certain expectations about finances—like who pays the bills, how money is shared, or who owns property—may be deeply ingrained. After heartbreak, you might find pressure from relatives to do things "the old way." Handling that:

- **Clarify Boundaries**: If family members try to interfere with your money decisions, gently but firmly let them know you appreciate their input but will handle things your way.

- **Educate Them If Possible**: Sometimes they worry due to lack of understanding. Explaining your budget or savings plan might ease their fears.
- **Stay True to Your Goals**: If you find their advice does not align with your long-term objectives, keep following your path politely.

Remember, it is your life. Other people's old traditions may not fit your current reality.

18. Finding Balance Between Self-Sufficiency and Healthy Support

Financial independence does not mean you have to do absolutely everything on your own if that leads to isolation or exhaustion:

- **Allow Healthy Support**: Accept help from trustworthy friends or family if it fits within a respectful relationship dynamic. Sometimes splitting rent with a roommate or living with family briefly can be a stepping stone.
- **Make Clear Agreements**: If someone offers to cover a certain bill, clarify whether it is a gift or a loan. Put it in writing if necessary, so misunderstandings do not arise later.
- **Reciprocate in Non-Financial Ways**: If someone helps you financially and you cannot pay them back with money, maybe you can offer childcare, cooking, or another form of assistance. Healthy support is about mutual respect, not feeling indebted or controlled.

Staying open to balanced cooperation ensures you do not burn out trying to prove independence overnight.

19. Acknowledging Financial Wins

When you reach a milestone—like paying off a credit card, saving a certain amount, or landing a better-paying job—take a moment to reflect on your hard work. This reflection can keep you motivated:

1. **Quiet Recognition**: Jot down the achievement in a journal to remind yourself later how far you have come.

2. **Small Reward**: If it fits your budget, buy a modest treat or enjoy a special meal at home. This is not about overspending but about marking progress.
3. **Share with a Trusted Friend**: Let someone supportive know about your achievement. Hearing them say, "Good job" can reinforce that you are moving in the right direction.

These simple acts can strengthen your resolve to keep improving your finances step by step.

---

20. The Link Between Financial Strength and Emotional Freedom

Ultimately, building financial independence is about creating a stable foundation for you to thrive emotionally. When money problems are in check:

- **You Feel Freer to Pursue Joy**: You can invest in hobbies, personal development, or travel without constant anxiety about bills.
- **Confidence in Relationships**: You are less likely to stay in a harmful situation due to financial need. You can choose connections based on love and mutual respect.
- **Healthier Coping**: With finances under control, you have more emotional space to focus on heartbreak recovery, therapy, or new friendships.

Money may not buy happiness, but it can remove obstacles that block your path to happiness. Achieving financial independence empowers you to build a more stable and fulfilling life, free from the weight of economic uncertainty.

---

21. Conclusion of Chapter 17

Financial independence is a crucial step toward emotional healing after heartbreak. By taking control of your income, expenses, and future planning, you can reduce stress and regain a sense of power over your life. Whether you start with a simple budget, tackle existing debts, or look for ways to grow your earning potential, each move away from financial dependence can spark new confidence in your ability to manage life's challenges.

As you work on your finances, remain mindful that it is a process, not an overnight fix. Small, consistent steps—paying off debt bit by bit, building an emergency fund, learning about investments—will gradually set you on solid ground. The freedom that comes from financial security gives you the emotional bandwidth to pursue healthier relationships and personal growth. In the next chapter, we will look at setting clear boundaries—a practice that can protect both your emotional and financial well-being, ensuring your progress is not undone by external pressures or unhealthy interactions.

Chapter 18: Setting Clear Boundaries

Healthy boundaries are essential for emotional stability, especially after heartbreak. Boundaries define how you interact with others, how much of your time and energy you give, and what behaviors you will not tolerate. Without them, you might get pulled back into old patterns or end up feeling overwhelmed by others' demands. This chapter will outline why boundaries matter, how to set them, and how to maintain them even when faced with pushback from people who preferred you without them.

1. Understanding What Boundaries Are

Boundaries are personal lines you create to protect your emotional space, values, and well-being. They tell others how to treat you and what you find acceptable or not acceptable in relationships. Boundaries can be physical, emotional, or digital:

- **Physical Boundaries**: Such as needing personal space, not wanting certain kinds of physical contact, or controlling who can enter your home.
- **Emotional Boundaries**: These deal with how much emotional energy you invest in someone, what topics you are willing to discuss, and how you want to be spoken to.
- **Digital Boundaries**: Relate to social media, texting frequency, and privacy settings—deciding how much access people have to your online life.

They serve as a guideline for healthy interactions, ensuring you do not become resentful or drained by other people's behavior.

2. Why Boundaries Are Crucial After Heartbreak

When a relationship ends, you might feel vulnerable. Old ties can linger, ex-partners might cross lines, or you might find yourself overly exposed to pressures from family and friends.

- **Prevent Emotional Exhaustion**: Protecting your mental energy ensures you have space to heal. If everyone dumps their opinions or demands on you, you might never find time to regroup.
- **Define a Fresh Start**: Setting new boundaries can mark a clear break from old habits that contributed to heartbreak.
- **Stop Unwanted Contact**: If your ex is texting or calling too much, boundaries help you decide if you want to respond, how often, or at all.

These reasons make boundary-setting a non-negotiable skill if you aim to recover and grow stronger.

3. Indicators You Need Stronger Boundaries

How do you know if your boundaries are weak or missing?

1. **Frequent Resentment**: You often feel upset about how people treat you, but you do not speak up.
2. **Excessive People-Pleasing**: You find yourself saying yes to requests even when you are exhausted or simply do not want to comply.
3. **Lack of Personal Space**: Others may show up unannounced, meddle in your private affairs, or text you constantly. You feel you cannot say no.
4. **Ongoing Conflict**: Repeated arguments might signal that you have not clearly stated your limits.

If these ring true, it is time to clarify your boundaries and enforce them.

4. Deciding Your Core Boundaries

Identifying where you stand on various issues helps you communicate your limits more effectively. Consider these categories:

- **Time**: How much time can you give to others each week? Which times of day do you prefer for calls or texts?
- **Emotional Labor**: Are you okay listening to a friend's problems daily, or do you need to limit how often you play therapist?
- **Personal Belongings**: Who can borrow your belongings? Under what conditions?

- **Privacy**: Do you want certain aspects of your life, like your finances or romantic status, to remain private?

Write these down to gain clarity. This list can grow or shift as your life changes.

---

5. Communicating Boundaries Firmly and Kindly

Once you know your boundaries, you must communicate them. The way you deliver your message affects how others respond.

1. **Use Clear Language**: Instead of hints or vague statements, be direct: "I need you to text me only once a day unless it is an emergency."
2. **Stay Calm**: Shouting or accusing can escalate tensions. Speak in a measured tone to show you are serious yet composed.
3. **Offer Brief Reasons**: You do not owe detailed explanations, but a short statement can help. For example, "I am focusing on my mental health," or "I have limited free time after work."

Clarity is key. People often test boundaries if they sense uncertainty or if the boundary is not stated plainly.

---

6. Examples of Simple Boundary Phrases

To make boundary-setting more concrete, here are examples you can use or adapt:

- **Time Boundary**: "I appreciate your need to talk, but I can only chat for 15 minutes tonight."
- **Emotional Boundary**: "I understand you are upset. However, I cannot continue this conversation if you use that tone."
- **Privacy Boundary**: "I am not comfortable sharing details about my personal finances right now."
- **Contact Boundary**: "I will respond to messages within 24 hours unless it is urgent."

These short statements are polite but firm, ensuring you convey your limit without inviting debate or personal attacks.

7. Handling Pushback or Guilt

People who benefited from your lack of boundaries might react poorly when you start setting them. Expect possible guilt trips or accusations of being cold or selfish:

- **Stand Firm**: Gently repeat your boundary if they continue to argue. "I hear you, but my position remains the same."
- **Resist Over-Explaining**: Too much justification can weaken your stance. You do not owe a detailed defense of your personal limit.
- **Release Undue Guilt**: You are not hurting anyone by drawing healthy lines. Another person's discomfort with your boundary does not mean you are wrong.

Pushback often comes from those who were used to you being more accommodating. Stay patient but unwavering.

8. Boundaries with an Ex-Partner

A breakup can leave many loose ends. If you want minimal contact, say so. If you must remain in contact (for example, co-parenting), define how that will happen:

- **Pick a Communication Method**: Maybe you prefer email or a specialized co-parenting app. This structure can keep emotional triggers low.
- **Set Topics**: Decide what you will talk about (children, shared property) and what is off-limits (personal opinions about each other's new relationships, etc.).
- **No Surprise Visits**: If your ex used to show up unannounced, clarify that they need permission or a set appointment. Lock doors if necessary.

By outlining these points, you create a sense of order that helps you heal without constant chaos.

9. Boundaries with Friends and Family

Sometimes family or close friends may believe they have free rein to intrude on your business, especially after heartbreak. While they may be well-meaning, you still have a right to privacy and respect:

1. **Limit Personal Questions**: If they probe into your dating status or finances, politely say, "I prefer not to talk about that."
2. **Mindful Visits**: If relatives show up without warning, propose that they call or text before coming over to ensure you are available.
3. **Control of Conversation**: Gently steer chatty friends away from painful subjects if you are not ready, or ask for a change of topic when it becomes too invasive.

Setting boundaries with loved ones can feel uncomfortable at first, but it ultimately leads to healthier connections.

---

10. Technology and Social Media Boundaries

Our digital lives can blur the lines between personal and public. Setting boundaries about your online presence can protect your peace:

- **Manage Friend Lists**: Remove or block your ex or negative influencers if their posts upset you.
- **Control Posting**: Avoid oversharing personal details that invite unsolicited advice or drama.
- **Set Communication Windows**: Decide times of day you will check messages or social media to prevent constant interruptions.

Digital boundaries help you maintain mental calm and reduce the risk of heartbreak triggers jumping out at you unannounced.

---

11. Emotional Boundaries at Work

After heartbreak, your personal life can seep into your work if you are not careful. Likewise, coworkers or supervisors might cross lines by prying into your situation:

1. **Draw a Line on Personal Topics**: You are not required to share details about your breakup or heartbreak with colleagues. A simple "I am handling some personal matters, but it is under control" can suffice.
2. **Avoid TMI**: Oversharing can lead to workplace gossip or discomfort.
3. **Focus on Tasks**: If a coworker keeps pushing you to talk, redirect the conversation back to work tasks or politely mention you would rather keep it professional.

Respecting your own privacy at work can keep heartbreak from undermining your professional life or reputation.

12. Learning to Say "No"

Saying no is one of the most direct ways to set boundaries:

- **Small Nos First**: Practice declining minor requests, like lending out your pen if you really do not want to. It might sound trivial, but it builds the habit of respecting your own wishes.
- **Use Polite Language**: "I appreciate you thinking of me, but I must decline this time."
- **Do Not Over-Explain**: A short statement is enough. Too much detail might invite arguments or attempts to change your mind.

Saying no is not rude if done calmly and politely. It is a self-care measure that prevents resentment and ensures you have time for what truly matters.

13. Self-Reflection and Boundaries

Setting boundaries is not just about telling others what to do. It also involves reflecting on your own behaviors:

- **Check for Mixed Signals**: Sometimes you might say, "Don't text me at night," but then you quickly reply to late-night messages. Consistent actions are vital for boundary enforcement.
- **Respect Others' Boundaries**: If you want your limits respected, reciprocate that respect in your relationships.

- **Update Boundaries Over Time**: As you heal from heartbreak and grow, certain boundaries may loosen or tighten. Review them periodically to ensure they still fit your life.

Boundaries are a two-way street: you hold others accountable, but you also respect the lines others set for themselves.

---

14. Signs a Boundary Is Being Violated

You might feel uneasy or get a gut feeling when a boundary is crossed:

1. **Sudden Anger or Anxiety**: An emotional spike might signal that someone just violated your comfort zone.
2. **Feeling Pressured**: If you sense you are being coerced into something that makes you uncomfortable, a boundary check is needed.
3. **Overstepping Patterns**: Repeated requests or actions that ignore what you have stated as your limit.

Do not ignore these signals. Address the issue promptly—calmly restating your boundary or, if necessary, removing yourself from the situation.

---

15. Maintaining Boundaries Under Stress

Life events—like heartbreak, job loss, or family emergencies—can weaken your resolve to keep boundaries, as you might feel needy or exhausted. Try these strategies:

- **Have a Reminder**: Write your core boundaries on a note in your phone or on a sticky note where you can see it.
- **Breathe Before Responding**: When stressed, you may impulsively say yes or drop your boundary to avoid conflict. A brief pause can help you stay true to your limits.
- **Seek Outside Input**: Talk to a supportive friend or counselor if you feel your boundary is slipping. They can reinforce why it is important.

Crisis times are when boundaries are tested, but also when they are most needed to protect your mental health.

16. Balancing Empathy with Firm Limits

Being empathetic and kind does not mean allowing others to walk all over you. You can care for others while holding your ground:

- **Express Understanding**: "I understand this is hard for you," followed by "but I still need you to respect my limit."
- **Validate Feelings**: Recognize their emotions without giving up your boundary. "I see you are upset, but I cannot lend you more money."
- **Offer Alternatives**: If someone wants more than you can give, suggest a middle path: "I can chat tomorrow for 15 minutes, but not tonight."

This method respects both your needs and the other person's feelings, preventing guilt from eroding your resolve.

---

17. When to Enforce Consequences

If someone repeatedly ignores your boundaries, consequences may be necessary to show you are serious. Consequences could be:

- **Reduced Interaction**: Limit how often you see or speak to the person who won't respect your boundaries.
- **End the Relationship**: In extreme cases, you might have to cut ties, especially if the violation is harmful or abusive.
- **Professional Support**: If there is harassment or stalking, contact authorities or legal counsel.

Consequences are not about punishing someone. They are about safeguarding your well-being when words alone fail.

---

18. Internal Boundaries

Sometimes the biggest boundary challenge is with yourself—resisting urges that harm your healing:

1. **Avoid Doom-Scrolling**: If checking your ex's social media triggers sadness or anger, set a personal rule to stop.

2. **Limit Negative Self-Talk**: Notice when you start berating yourself and choose a kinder approach.
3. **Protect Your Time**: Plan your day so you do not waste hours on activities that do not match your goals or values.

By honoring the limits you set for your own behavior, you reinforce self-respect and stability.

---

19. Recognizing Growth Through Boundaries

As you strengthen your boundaries, watch for positive signs:

- **Increased Self-Confidence**: You start to trust your own instincts and decisions, rather than needing external validation.
- **Better Relationships**: Friends and family might respect you more, leading to healthier, more equal dynamics.
- **Less Overwhelm**: You feel calmer, with fewer emotional rollercoasters triggered by others' actions.

These changes show that boundaries are not walls shutting out love. Instead, they are frameworks that allow love, respect, and understanding to flourish without chaos.

---

20. Making Boundaries a Lasting Practice

Boundaries are not a one-time fix; they are an ongoing habit. Keep them strong by:

1. **Regular Check-Ins**: Every month or so, ask yourself if any boundary is being tested.
2. **Stay Flexible**: Some boundaries might become less critical over time, or new ones might become necessary.
3. **Celebrate Progress**: Each time you successfully enforce a boundary, take a mental note of how it feels to stand up for yourself.

Acknowledging your growth keeps you motivated to maintain the boundaries that protect your new emotional stability.

21. Conclusion of Chapter 18

Setting clear boundaries is a powerful step to protect your emotional recovery after heartbreak. By defining what you will and will not tolerate, you create a safer environment for healing and growth. Boundaries can be physical, emotional, or digital, and they apply to everyone—ex-partners, friends, family, coworkers, and even yourself.

Though you might face resistance, especially from people used to having unlimited access to your time or emotions, standing firm in your limits helps you avoid repeating old patterns of hurt or resentment. Each boundary you set and maintain strengthens your sense of self-worth and your ability to nurture healthy, respectful relationships moving forward.

With your finances and boundaries in order, you are well on your way to a more secure and balanced life. In the next chapters, we will address finding purpose outside romantic love and building a future that aligns with your true self. Step by step, you can create a life that honors your emotional well-being, free from the chaos of past heartbreak and guided by the structure of caring yet firm boundaries.

Chapter 19: Finding Purpose Outside Romantic Love

Romantic love can feel like a central pillar in many people's lives, especially if they have been in a long-term relationship or if they have always placed significant importance on partnership. After heartbreak, it is common to feel disoriented or unsure about what direction to take. However, there is much more to a person's identity than the role they play in a romantic bond. This chapter will explore how to discover or rediscover meaningful purposes outside of romantic ties. This can help rebuild confidence, spark creativity, and bring a renewed sense of direction that does not rely solely on one's romantic status.

---

1. Why Purpose Outside Romantic Love Matters

1. **Personal Identity**: A person is more than a partner or a spouse. Recognizing your individuality supports healthier self-esteem and reduces the chance of codependency.
2. **Emotional Stability**: Having multiple interests or goals provides a cushion when heartbreak hits. If one aspect of your life falters, other parts remain intact, giving you emotional resilience.
3. **Long-Term Growth**: Focusing on personal visions often triggers new achievements, skills, or insights. These can shape a future in which relationships are one fulfilling aspect, not the entire picture.

Understanding that love is just one chapter of a multifaceted life can relieve the pressure to find immediate closure in romance. It opens doors to new explorations of who you are.

---

2. Recognizing Different Areas of Life

When a breakup happens, it is easy to dwell on the loss of companionship. But broadening your vision to various life domains can help you see that you have other areas to tend to:

- **Career and Work**: Whether it is a job or a long-term career path, these tasks can offer structure and a chance to build expertise.

- **Hobbies and Interests**: Activities unrelated to romance can feed creativity, intellect, or physical health.
- **Social Connections**: Friendships, community involvement, and family bonds can provide support and camaraderie.
- **Personal Well-Being**: Spiritual practices (if relevant), mental health, and physical health are pillars of a balanced life.

Looking at life as a collection of spheres reminds you that losing one sphere (a romantic relationship) does not mean everything else is gone.

---

3. The Concept of Core Values

Core values are the guiding principles that shape your behavior and priorities. They act like a compass in life:

1. **Identifying Your Values**: Consider words or ideas that matter most to you: honesty, adventure, learning, generosity, creativity, stability, etc.
2. **Aligning Activities**: Check if your daily habits reflect those values. If creativity is important but you never engage in artistic projects, perhaps it is time to adjust.
3. **Using Values for Decision-Making**: Values can guide your next moves. For example, if compassion is central, volunteering or helping others might be a path to greater purpose.

These values often remain consistent, with some evolving over time. By revisiting them after heartbreak, you can find stable ground and a sense of meaning unrelated to romantic status.

---

4. Pursuing Personal Passions

Many individuals enter relationships and gradually reduce time for personal passions. A breakup may highlight how those interests were set aside. Reconnecting with them can bring fresh excitement:

- **Revisit Old Hobbies**: Think back to what you loved doing before the relationship. Perhaps you used to bake, do crosswords, study languages, or play an instrument. Start small—maybe 30 minutes a week—and let the enjoyment grow.

- **Try New Skills**: If old hobbies do not resonate anymore, sample something new. Join a dance class, learn a programming language, or take up knitting. This ignites curiosity and can help you discover hidden talents.
- **Share With Others**: Sometimes practicing passions with a group or club intensifies the experience. It also provides potential for making new friends.

Exploring or revisiting hobbies can remind you that you have unique skills and preferences that exist independently of any partner.

---

5. Volunteering and Community Service

One potent way to find purpose is by helping others. Offering your skills or time to a worthy cause can foster a sense of fulfillment and connection:

1. **Community Projects**: Local animal shelters, food banks, or environmental cleanups might need volunteers. This direct interaction can show you tangible results of your efforts.
2. **Online Volunteering**: If in-person volunteering is tough, virtual options exist for tutoring, crisis hotlines, or nonprofit administration tasks.
3. **Skill-Based Service**: If you have a specific skill—like graphic design, accounting, or teaching—a charitable organization might benefit from it.

Engaging in service can shift attention away from heartbreak, reduce self-focused rumination, and build a sense of contribution to a bigger picture.

---

6. Exploring Spiritual or Philosophical Interests

Some people find purpose in exploring beliefs about life, the universe, or human nature. This can be religious or non-religious:

- **Meditation and Mindfulness**: Practices that encourage calm observation of thoughts can bring clarity and deeper self-awareness.
- **Religious Communities**: If you have a faith tradition, attending gatherings or speaking with spiritual leaders might offer a broader sense of belonging.

- **Philosophical Study**: Reading works of famous thinkers can spark contemplation about ethics, purpose, and how to live a meaningful life.

These inquiries can provide comfort and a sense that your life has depth beyond romantic pursuits, giving you a new framework for seeing yourself and your role in the world.

---

7. Building a Life Mission Statement

Some individuals find it useful to craft a personal mission statement—a concise summary of what you want to stand for:

1. **Reflect on Long-Term Desires**: Ask yourself how you want to be remembered, what change you want to see in yourself or the world, and what truly excites you.
2. **Phrase It Clearly**: Keep it short and focused. For example, "I aim to bring warmth and creativity to those around me through teaching, art, and supportive friendships."
3. **Revisit Often**: Print it or save it on your phone. Checking it when you feel lost can keep you grounded.

A mission statement does not have to be final or perfect. It is just a guiding reference for personal priorities, especially helpful when heartbreak triggers questions about life direction.

---

8. Healthy Relationship with Work and Goals

Be careful that seeking purpose does not lead to overwork or ignoring emotional needs. Sometimes heartbreak can push people to bury themselves in professional tasks:

- **Avoid Burnout**: While focusing on a career can be fulfilling, working excessive hours to sidestep emotional pain might create health or stress problems later.
- **Set Achievable Objectives**: Make sure your professional goals are realistic. Celebrate small progress toward them.

- **Create Work-Life Balance**: Even if single, you deserve time to rest, socialize, and pursue interests. A balanced routine helps maintain emotional well-being.

Moderation is key. A strong sense of purpose in work can be beneficial, but not if it replaces all other aspects of life or compounds heartbreak stress.

---

9. Turning Past Pain into Personal Growth

Heartbreak can act as a catalyst for transformation. Beyond simply "moving on," you can look at what insights or motivations the breakup offers:

1. **Lessons Learned**: Perhaps you discovered the kind of behaviors you will no longer accept or recognized you had neglected certain parts of yourself.
2. **Fuel for Future Endeavors**: Pain can be repurposed into energy for writing a book, launching a passion project, or supporting others undergoing heartbreak.
3. **Inspiring Change**: If the relationship ended over a mutual problem, you might adopt a new attitude or habits that better match your real identity.

Using heartbreak as a spark can lead you to create something meaningful, be it an improved lifestyle or a community initiative.

---

10. Embracing Creativity

Creativity often brings a sense of flow, where you lose track of time because you are fully immersed in the activity. This can serve as a powerful form of self-discovery:

- **Artistic Expression**: Painting, sketching, photography, or even adult coloring books can channel emotions in a constructive way.
- **Writing**: Journaling, poetry, or blogging about topics you care about can clarify your thoughts and generate new ideas about life's possibilities.
- **Music and Performance**: Learning an instrument or taking part in local theater groups can connect you to a community of enthusiasts.

Channeling heartbreak energy into creative tasks transforms pain into expressions that can lighten emotional burdens.

11. Strengthening Friendships and Social Circles

Romantic love often gets top billing in many lives, overshadowing friendships. A heartbreak can reveal the value of non-romantic ties:

1. **Connect Regularly**: Schedule calls, coffee meets, or walks with friends. Genuine bonds grow through consistency and sharing experiences.
2. **Mutual Support**: Offer help to friends who might also be dealing with issues. The reciprocal nature of supportive friendships enhances belonging.
3. **Host Gatherings**: Bring people together for casual get-togethers, game nights, or skill-sharing events. This can create a sense of community.

Friendships are a reminder that you are not alone and that affection and support exist outside romantic contexts.

12. Physical Well-Being as a Source of Purpose

Focusing on physical health can restore self-esteem and create a routine that brings a sense of accomplishment:

- **Exercise Routines**: Whether jogging, yoga-like stretching, or weight training, consistent physical activity helps mood, confidence, and bodily health.
- **Nutrition**: Cooking healthy meals can be a purposeful habit, letting you experiment with recipes and take care of your body.
- **Outdoor Adventures**: Hiking, bicycling, or simply exploring parks fosters a connection with nature. This can be calming and mentally refreshing.

A stable physical regimen can ground your life in healthy habits that do not depend on a partner's encouragement or participation.

13. Expanding Your Knowledge and Skills

Lifelong learning, whether formal or informal, provides a sense of progress:

1. **Take Classes**: Community centers or online platforms offer classes in languages, coding, culinary arts, or crafts.
2. **Attend Workshops**: Seminars on personal finance, leadership, or creative writing can add new layers to your abilities.
3. **Self-Study**: Books, podcasts, and documentaries let you explore interests at your own pace.

This intellectual growth shows you that your mind can keep evolving, a reminder that life's possibilities do not end with a romantic breakup.

---

14. Travel or Local Exploration

Sometimes experiencing fresh environments can shift your perspective. This does not require going halfway around the globe; local exploration also works:

- **Weekend Trips**: Short visits to nearby towns or natural attractions can re-energize you and spark curiosity.
- **Culture and Museums**: Art exhibitions, historical museums, or science centers can expand your worldview and inspire new thoughts about your place in the world.
- **Solo Travel**: It can be intimidating at first, but traveling alone fosters independence, problem-solving, and confidence.

Stepping away from familiar surroundings, even briefly, can highlight aspects of yourself that you rarely notice in everyday routines.

---

15. Considering Mentorship or Coaching Roles

If you have accumulated experiences—professionally or personally—you might find purpose in guiding others:

1. **Professional Mentoring**: In your workplace or industry, you could help newcomers or interns. Sharing knowledge can remind you of your own competencies.

2. **Life Skills Mentoring**: If you overcame obstacles such as heartbreak or financial struggles, you might offer advice or moral support to those going through similar challenges.
3. **Community Programs**: Libraries, youth centers, or local organizations often seek mentors for children or teenagers who need positive role models.

Mentoring underscores that personal struggles, including heartbreak, can be turned into wisdom that benefits others.

16. Building Self-Trust

A key component in finding purpose is trusting your own judgment and abilities. Heartbreak can shake this trust. Rebuilding it involves:

- **Reflecting on Past Successes**: Recall times you solved problems or succeeded at tasks without leaning on a romantic partner.
- **Giving Yourself Credit**: When you handle a new project or make a positive decision, note it in a journal or a notes app.
- **Practicing Self-Compassion**: Accept that mistakes or misjudgments may happen. Rather than condemning yourself, treat these moments as part of the learning curve.

As self-trust grows, you can pursue new aims without excessive fear of failure, because you believe in your resilience.

17. Setting Small Challenges

Challenges can invigorate your sense of purpose, breaking monotony and reminding you of your capacity to grow:

1. **Physical Challenges**: A 5K race, a home exercise routine, or climbing a small mountain if physically able.
2. **Creative Challenges**: A 30-day writing challenge, daily sketches, or weekly photography tasks.
3. **Personal Development Goals**: Reading a certain number of books, learning to cook a new dish every week, or budgeting consistently for a month.

Small achievements add up. They show you that life can advance in meaningful ways, independent of romantic involvement.

18. Managing External Pressures About Love

Society, family, and friends sometimes push the idea that romantic partnership is essential for a complete life. That pressure can distract from personal growth:

- **Politely Redirect**: If someone asks, "Why are you still single?" respond by mentioning a goal or project you are excited about.
- **Limit Exposure**: If certain social media accounts or acquaintances make you feel bad for not being in a relationship, reduce time spent on them.
- **Affirm Your Choices**: Remind yourself that stepping away from romance for a while can be intentional and healthy.

You have the right to define your own version of a worthwhile life, with or without a partner.

19. Overcoming Internalized Expectations

Beyond external pressure, individuals often carry internal scripts like "I should be married by 30" or "I am incomplete without a partner." Confronting these beliefs can open the door to genuine self-discovery:

1. **Question the Script**: Ask where the expectation came from—family tradition, media, or cultural norms? Are these relevant to you now?
2. **Redefine Success**: If you previously measured success by relationship milestones, consider alternative measures: personal achievements, creative outputs, or community contributions.
3. **Therapeutic Support**: A counselor can help identify deep-seated beliefs and guide you to replace them with healthier definitions of self-worth.

Dismantling these internal pressures frees you to discover a life purpose not dictated by relationship status.

20. Balancing Independence with Openness to Future Love

Finding purpose outside romance does not mean rejecting the idea of love forever. Rather, it means not relying on it as the sole anchor. You can hold these two truths:

- **It Is Okay to Desire a Future Relationship**: Being open to love down the line can coexist with building a rich, self-driven life right now.
- **You Are Already Whole**: Whether single or partnered, you remain a complete person with valid talents, dreams, and value. A relationship can enhance your life, but not define it entirely.

This balance helps avoid extremes—neither fixating on romance as the only goal nor completely dismissing the possibility of future connections.

---

21. Conclusion of Chapter 19

Finding purpose beyond romantic love expands your identity, allowing you to live a fuller life that does not hinge on any single relationship. By engaging in meaningful work, developing personal passions, cultivating friendships, and exploring your own values, you build a robust sense of self. Heartbreak can then become an event that triggered positive self-discovery instead of a permanent limitation.

This approach does not deny the pain of losing someone you cared about. However, it turns that pain into a stepping stone toward deeper fulfillment. By seeking purpose in various areas—career, hobbies, community, health, spirituality—you create multiple pillars of support. When one pillar is shaken, the others stand firm. With a solid sense of identity and value, you become more resilient and open to life's possibilities.

In the final chapter, we will focus on moving forward with hope and strength. We will explore how to keep bitterness from overshadowing future experiences, how to maintain a balanced outlook on love, and how to enter new phases of life without the baggage of heartbreak dragging you down.

Chapter 20: Moving Forward with Hope and Strength

This is the concluding chapter, tying together all the insights and methods discussed throughout the book. Heartbreak can leave scars, but it can also mark the start of positive change. Having addressed the emotional effects, self-care basics, the importance of reaching out for support, rebuilding trust, handling physical symptoms, creating financial independence, and setting boundaries, you are now in a position to move forward. Here, we will examine practical ways to maintain hope and inner strength, so that your life remains meaningful and fulfilling, no matter what happened in the past.

---

1. Accepting the Reality of Change

One of the biggest sources of pain after a breakup is fighting reality—wishing the relationship had not ended or that events had turned out differently. Accepting change does not equal liking it, but it does help you move on:

- **Acknowledge Impermanence**: Recognize that many things in life—jobs, friendships, romantic ties—might be temporary. This does not diminish their value; it simply places them in perspective.
- **Focus on the Present**: Instead of reliving regrets, direct your attention to what you can influence right now: your habits, your environment, your goals for the next few weeks.
- **Learn from the Past**: Reflect on lessons, but do not dwell on "if only." Transformation often starts once you accept that some chapters have closed.

This shift can free mental space for positive planning, letting your energy flow into building a bright future rather than clinging to a shattered dream.

---

2. Guarding Against Cynicism

After a painful experience, some people develop a cynical outlook, believing that love leads only to hurt or that people are untrustworthy. Though understandable, cynicism can limit your capacity for joy and connection:

1. **Recognize Bitterness**: When you notice thoughts like "All relationships fail eventually," understand it may be a defense mechanism protecting you from future pain.
2. **Balance Realism with Openness**: Accept that heartbreak can happen, but also acknowledge that sincere bonds and supportive friendships exist.
3. **Stay Curious**: Challenge blanket statements with questions: "Is it truly all relationships that fail?" "Have I not seen any healthy relationships around me?" This approach keeps cynicism from becoming your default mindset.

Retaining hope does not make you naive; it allows you to stay open to possibilities of growth and happiness in all areas of life.

---

3. Cultivating Self-Compassion

The healing process after heartbreak can include moments of guilt or self-blame, especially if you recall regrets from the relationship. Offering compassion to yourself fosters better emotional resilience:

- **Speak Kindly to Yourself**: Imagine talking to a dear friend who feels at fault. How would you comfort them? Use similar words on your own behalf.
- **Accept Imperfection**: Recognize you are human. Dwelling on "I should have done better" prolongs suffering. Instead, note the lessons and move forward.
- **Counter Negative Thoughts**: When your mind floods with self-criticism, actively replace it with balanced viewpoints: "I made errors, but I am learning. I can treat myself with understanding."

Self-compassion reduces emotional burdens and fosters patience during the ups and downs of moving on.

---

4. Building Emotional Strength Through Daily Habits

Long-term recovery often depends on small, consistent habits that boost mental resilience:

1. **Morning Routine**: A short practice like five minutes of calm breathing, journaling, or stretching sets a stable tone for the day.
2. **Set Micro-Goals**: Whether it is completing a chapter of a book, cooking a healthy meal, or organizing a small part of your living space, achieving tiny targets can lift your mood.
3. **Evening Reflection**: Spend a minute or two noting what went well or what you appreciate. This trains your mind to spot positive elements rather than focusing on heartbreak alone.

Emotional strength, like physical strength, grows from repeated, modest exercises over time.

---

5. Reentry Into the Social World

As you heal, you might feel ready to attend gatherings or meet potential new friends or partners. Approaching social situations with a balanced mindset can help:

- **Pace Yourself**: If large parties are overwhelming, opt for smaller meetups or casual coffee dates. Gradual exposure to social circles rebuilds your comfort.
- **Stay Genuine**: Resist pretending everything is perfect if you still feel raw. You do not have to spill all details, but a touch of honesty—"I am going through a personal transition right now"—can keep things authentic.
- **Respect Personal Readiness**: If you are not ready to date seriously, do not force it because of external pressure. On the other hand, if you do feel ready, do not let fear hold you back unnecessarily.

Balancing vulnerability with self-awareness lets you gradually expand your social horizons without jeopardizing emotional stability.

---

6. Introducing Hope in Your Thought Patterns

Hope is more than blind optimism. It involves believing that improvement is possible and that you can influence positive outcomes:

1. **Use "What If" Positively**: Instead of "What if I fail?" ask "What if things turn out better than I think?"

2. **Collect Real-Life Examples**: Look for people who overcame heartbreak or adversity. Their stories can remind you that hardship does not last forever.
3. **Future-Oriented Thinking**: Imagine yourself six months or a year from now, feeling stronger, exploring new projects, or deepening supportive friendships.

Even small glimpses of hope can diffuse despair and give you momentum to keep trying.

7. Handling Relapses or Emotional Setbacks

Healing from heartbreak is rarely linear. You might have days or weeks of feeling strong, only to face a wave of sadness or frustration. This is normal:

- **View Setbacks as Part of the Process**: Accept that emotional dips do not erase prior progress. They are often signals that you need rest or reflection.
- **Identify Triggers**: Maybe a certain place, song, or social media post stirs up old memories. Recognizing triggers can help you plan how to respond next time.
- **Practice Kindness**: Instead of blaming yourself for "not being over it yet," acknowledge that healing is layered and can reemerge in phases.

By responding to relapses with understanding, you avoid harsh self-judgment that can prolong emotional pain.

8. Evaluating Your Growth

Actively reviewing your improvements can reinforce a sense of progress:

1. **Ask Key Questions**: "Have I learned new coping skills since the breakup?" "Am I more aware of red flags?" "Do I handle conflicts differently now?"
2. **Compare Mindsets**: Reflect on how you felt right after heartbreak and how you feel today. Even small shifts in optimism or confidence count.
3. **Acknowledge Achievements**: Whether you gained new friends, handled finances better, or started a creative project, these are signs of forward movement.

This evaluation helps you see that heartbreak was not the end; it became a pivot point for self-improvement.

9. Embracing a Philosophy of Trial and Error

Life after heartbreak often involves experimentation—trying new routines, meeting new people, or tackling different hobbies. Sometimes these steps will not go as planned:

- **Keep Expectations Moderate**: Not every new adventure will yield remarkable results, but each attempt teaches you something.
- **Laugh at Small Mishaps**: If you discover a hobby you dislike or a social event that is dull, treat it as an amusing learning experience rather than a personal failure.
- **Avoid Perfectionism**: Accepting that not everything will be perfect frees you to explore without crippling fear of making mistakes.

Viewing life as a series of attempts and lessons prevents heartbreak from stalling your willingness to try fresh opportunities.

10. Healthy Approaches to Future Relationships

Moving on with hope does not necessarily require jumping into a new romance, but eventually, you might be open to it. To approach it wisely:

1. **Check Self-Readiness**: Are you able to consider a new partner without obsessing over your ex or carrying unresolved anger? A bit of leftover sadness is normal, but strong bitterness may signal you need more time.
2. **Maintain Boundaries**: Lessons from previous chapters about boundaries remain relevant in new connections.
3. **Communicate Honestly**: If you do meet someone, share your emotional position at a comfortable pace, ensuring they understand you are recovering but not helpless.

Moving forward does not mean forgetting the past entirely. It means carrying lessons that foster healthier patterns and a measured approach to trust.

11. Sustaining Long-Term Hope

Hope can fade if not occasionally replenished. Some strategies for keeping a hopeful mindset:

- **Regular Inspiration**: Follow social media accounts, podcasts, or newsletters that share uplifting stories or motivational ideas.
- **Create Visual Reminders**: A vision board or a collage of quotes can remind you each day of the direction you aim for.
- **Share Hope with Others**: Encourage friends in their pursuits. Being supportive can also reinforce your own positivity.

Hope thrives in an environment of shared encouragement and personal reflection. Keeping it alive ensures heartbreak does not cast a permanent shadow over your life's outlook.

---

12. Combining Self-Reflection with Action

While introspection is important, action solidifies growth. If you always stay in your head, heartbreak might remain theoretical:

- **Balanced Lifestyle**: Pair self-reflection time (like journaling or therapy) with practical steps (applying for a class, starting an exercise routine).
- **Self-Care in Motion**: Sometimes the best healing happens while doing tasks—like painting, hiking, reorganizing your space—rather than sitting still.
- **Goal Checkpoints**: If you set a goal (writing 500 words daily, volunteering monthly), schedule periodic reviews to see how you are doing.

This balanced approach stops rumination from stalling you while still allowing thoughtful analysis of emotional progress.

---

13. Recognizing That Strength Can Be Quiet

A common misconception is that moving on with "strength" means always being loud, bold, or outwardly confident. Strength can also be subtle:

- **Gentle Endurance**: The act of waking up every day and doing small tasks consistently, even with a heavy heart, is a form of bravery.
- **Silent Determination**: Making tough choices—like cutting off toxic ties or dedicating time to a personal mission—without fanfare still requires courage.
- **Respecting Limits**: Knowing when to rest or ask for help also shows inner fortitude, as it reveals self-awareness rather than stubbornness.

Strength does not always roar. Sometimes it exists in the quiet confidence of someone who refuses to give up on their life's potential, even after heartbreak.

---

14. Giving Back to Those Around You

A hopeful outlook often expands to caring for others. Contributing to someone else's well-being can further reinforce your own sense of purpose:

- **Small Acts of Kindness**: Compliment a coworker's efforts, help a neighbor with groceries, or check in on a friend who might be lonely.
- **Community Service**: Building on the volunteering discussion from earlier chapters, ongoing service can maintain perspective on life's bigger picture.
- **Peer Support**: Sharing how you managed heartbreak might comfort someone facing a fresh breakup. You become an example that pain does not last forever.

Focusing on others can be a healthy step, as it balances personal healing with outward empathy, preventing self-absorption during a tough emotional period.

---

15. Letting Go of Comparisons

When you see others who seem to have smoothly found new love or appear fully recovered, you might feel inadequate. But each person's timeline and process differ:

- **Recognize Surface Impressions**: Online posts or casual acquaintances do not always show hidden struggles.
- **Revisit Your Own Goals**: Keep your eyes on your own path, trusting that genuine progress often takes quiet, consistent effort.

- **Honor Your Unique Path**: If you take longer to heal or want to remain single for a while, it is valid. Resist the urge to judge your life based on someone else's highlight reel.

Comparisons can drain hope and spark envy. Shifting focus to your personal progress fosters peaceful acceptance of your place in life.

16. Monitoring Your Inner Circle

The people you regularly interact with can shape your attitude toward life:

1. **Encouraging Companions**: Seek those who respect your healing pace, support your new interests, and avoid shaming you about heartbreak.
2. **Healthy Challenges**: Good friends might gently challenge negative self-talk or push you to step out of comfort zones.
3. **Stepping Away from Toxicity**: If certain individuals belittle your growth or constantly drag your mood down, limit your exposure.

Surrounding yourself with a supportive network can multiply your own strength and hope, creating a feedback loop of positivity.

17. Reinventing Personal Rituals

Certain rituals, once shared with an ex, might cause sadness—such as Sunday brunch or nightly calls. Instead of lamenting these lost routines, craft new personal or social rituals:

- **Solo Evening Ritual**: A calming bath with soft music, reading a favorite book, or reflecting on daily gratitude.
- **Weekly Meetups with Friends**: A standing coffee date or group video call can fill the gap of old relationship habits.
- **Creative Projects**: Start a "Sunday creation session" where you paint, write, or build something, turning what was once a couples' tradition into a personal creative time.

By replacing old traditions, you reclaim those slots in your life and fill them with fresh meaning.

18. Long-Term View: Life Beyond Heartbreak

A practical exercise is to imagine yourself years down the road, well past heartbreak:

- **Ask "Where Do I See Myself?"**: Consider the kind of person you want to be, the environment you hope to create, and the relationships you want to maintain.
- **Brainstorm Next Steps**: Look at how you can steer daily decisions so they match that envisioned future.
- **Acknowledge Flexibility**: The future might not unfold exactly as you plan, but having a direction can inspire consistent moves that shape your reality.

Thinking long-term reminds you that heartbreak is not the final chapter. It is an event that, while significant, does not define your entire life story.

---

19. Giving Yourself Time to Heal

Media often glorifies quick bounce-backs, but true emotional strength develops at its own pace:

- **Resist Rushing**: You do not need to "get over it" on someone else's timetable. If it takes months or more, that is okay.
- **Be Patient with Emotions**: Some days you might feel confident, while others you might feel lonely. These fluctuations are part of the process.
- **Celebrate Glimpses of Peace**: Even a momentary sense of relief or lightness is a sign that healing is in progress.

Healing is a personal timeline, so giving yourself permission to move at your natural speed is an act of self-respect.

---

20. Crafting Your Narrative

Each person has a personal narrative about their heartbreak. Rewriting that narrative can shift you from victimhood to empowerment:

- **Identify the Old Story**: "I was abandoned," "I am unlucky in love," or "I failed at relationships."
- **Rewrite the Script**: "I faced a painful chapter, but I learned to stand up for my needs," or "I discovered new strengths I never knew I had."
- **Live by the New Story**: Let this revised perspective guide how you talk about the past and how you envision the future.

Reframing heartbreak as part of your growth story, rather than a crippling event, positions you to move forward with a sense of triumph over adversity.

---

21. Conclusion of Chapter 20

Moving forward with hope and strength after heartbreak is a multifaceted process. It involves accepting what has changed, guarding against cynicism, holding onto your self-worth, and gradually re-entering the world of social connections. You learn to integrate the lessons from past pain, rather than allowing them to define your destiny. With consistent self-reflection and gentle progress, you can release bitterness and keep your heart open to new possibilities.

By staying mindful of your boundaries, focusing on personal growth and purposeful living, and cherishing the supportive network around you, you reclaim ownership of your life. Heartbreak becomes a part of your story—a meaningful chapter that, while painful, set in motion transformations you might never have initiated otherwise. With hope lighting your way, you step confidently into each new day, trusting that you carry the resilience to face what comes, and the strength to continue building a fulfilling future on your terms.

This completes our exploration of heartbreak, healing, and empowerment. You now have tools to handle pain, rebuild self-worth, set financial and emotional boundaries, nurture friendships, and find purpose outside romantic love. Most importantly, you have the capacity to proceed with a renewed sense of hope and inner strength, ready to shape a life that honors who you are, heartbreak or not.

www.ingramcontent.com/pod-product-compliance
Lightning Source LLC
LaVergne TN
LVHW012105070526
838202LV00056B/5632